Sensual
SOUL SHINE

Sensual SOUL SHINE

the Reclamation *of the* Feminine

created by
Women Who Live Sensually

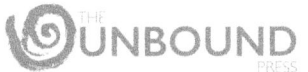

Copyright © 2024 by Carrie Myers

All rights reserved. No part of this publication may be reproduced, distributed or transmitted in anyform or by any means without permission of the publisher, except in the case of brief quotations referencing the body of work and in accordance with copyright law.

The information given in this book should not be treated as a substitute for professional medical advice; always consult a medical practitioner. Any use of information in this book is at the reader's discretion and risk. Neither the author nor the publisher can be held responsible for any loss, claim or damage arising out of the use, or misuse, of the suggestions made, the failure to take medical advice of for any material on third party websites.

Original cover art: Kelsey Wyatt

ISBN 978-1-916529-17-5 Paperback
ISBN 978-1-916529-18-2 Ebook

The Unbound Press
www.theunboundpress.com

Hey unbound one!

Welcome to this magical book brought to you by The Unbound Press.

At The Unbound Press we believe that when women write freely from the fullest expression of who they are, it can't help but activate a feeling of deep connection and transformation in others. When we come together, we become more and we're changing the world, one book at a time!

This book has been carefully crafted by both the contributors and publisher with the intention of inspiring you to move ever more deeply into who you truly are.

We hope that this book helps you to connect with your Unbound Self and that you feel called to pass it on to others who want to live a more fully expressed life.

With much love,
Nicola Humber

Founder of The Unbound Press

www.theunboundpress.com

This book is dedicated to women all over the world, who have come out from the shadows and are living in their sensual, authentic, feminine selves.

This book is the journey of the women who have decided to leave traumas, social constructs, rules, and expectations behind to ReClaim their radiant, authentic, feminine, and sensual selves. As you read the words of these brave women, let them inspire you to take control of your life, your destiny, your pleasure, and your wholeness as a woman.

Reclaiming your feminine is like a deep sigh of relief as we step into a space of authenticity within ourselves. As we release the strong masculine societal expectations, we allow our flow to be intuitive, easeful, nurturing, and meaningful.

Are you ready to venture into your soul, fully claiming who you have always been meant to be?

CONTENTS

Foreword - Heather Iden - xiii

1. Remember Your Inner Little Girl - Carrie Myers — 1
2. Define Your Sensuality - Carrie Myers — 3
3. Pacing Behind the Gate - Carrie Myers — 5
4. What IS Sensuality? - Carrie Myers — 7
5. Curiosity, Imagination and Sensuality - Carrie Myers — 11
6. Skinny Dip & Succumb - Annette Vaucanson Kelly — 17
7. Remembering My Sensual, Soulful Self - Katie May — 29
8. The Good and Sexy Vietnamese Woman - Elizabeth Nguyen — 37
9. The Masculine and Feminine Take a Hike - Carrie Myers — 47
10. Reclaim Your Sensuality With Nature - Carrie Myers — 49
11. Finding Sensuality in the Masculine World - Carrie Myers — 53
12. Living Life Wide Open - Heather Robbins — 57
13. Love Notes to Me, From the Depths of My Soul - Katie Weiper — 65
14. Burning Down the House - Kim Lange (Huynh) — 77
15. Suppressing the Sensual for Safety - Carrie Myers — 91
16. Woman On Fire - Carrie Myers — 96
17. She Said Connection - Carrie Myers — 97
18. The Pleasure Practice - Laurie Riedman — 99
19. Homecoming - Nicola Humber — 109
20. Your Authentic Expression - Patricia Alessandra Levy — 121
21. Unshackled: A Return to Erotic Innocence - Siobhan Gannon — 139
22. My Sensual Circle - Carrie Myers — 159
23. Grab Your Journal - Carrie Myers — 165

About the Lead Author - Carrie Myers - 173

FOREWORD
by Heather Iden

I met Carrie at a time in my life where darkness had settled in for both of us, a time of very fragile sensuality and sense of self. We had instant karma, and each recognized the strength they had to offer the other. Our friendship supported healing and growth. I have been fortunate enough to witness Carrie's journey as she shares her gifts with the world.

Along the way, Carrie recognized the community of women today was lacking or interrupted by the pace and race of life and it stirred the light within her. I watched her bloom. She used yoga, poetry, self-development, and writing. Such a journey is often a winding road rather than a straight path. By inviting women to discuss, write about, and let go on the mat, a clear theme beat at the heart of many women. What is it to be feminine today and how can we stand in it? Can we embrace what we feel in the pit of our stomachs: the maiden, mother, and crone? Is there a right way to embrace the feminine?

This book is her work of building a feminine community around sensuality, feminine sensuality. Embracing the pleasure of the feminine and discovering the magic created when the stillness of a heartbeat bursts at the seams in warm waves. Learning that female pleasure isn't selfish, rather the activation of a magic as old as time. Remembering that our voices and bodies are full of healing and wisdom.

The women in this book reveal the hills and valleys in discovering your feminine and embracing the ebb and flow that is womanhood. The diverse stories demonstrate the impact of so many things on female sensuality and feature the ultimate power of choice we all have.

The power lies within. Enjoy the journey.

REMEMBER YOUR INNER LITTLE GIRL

by Carrie Myers

As little girls, we danced in the meadows with crowns of flowers adorning our hair. As we grew and walked from those meadows full of inspiration and sunshine, we began collecting thorns and muck that wilted our flower crowns, blocked our glow, our shine, and our unique, sensual selves. We dimmed so subtly that we barely realize we are almost extinguished.

ReClaim your magic as you flow through the pages of **Sensual Soul Shine.**

You may want to invest in a beautiful journal and new pen to take notes on the wisdom that you read and on the wisdom that you discover from within.

'What is your definition of sensuality, as you begin this book? Then come back to this question as you finish it. See how your definition changes, grows, and expands.'

— Carrie Myers

Define Your Sensuality
by Carrie Myers

I was going to start this book out with a dictionary definition of *sensuality*, but as I was looking through the definitions, none of them seemed to embody the full spectrum of *sensuality*. So, I decided that I would let you come to your own conclusion of the definition of *sensuality*, because it means something different for each woman. The feeling, the authenticity, the movement, the confidence, and the look of *sensuality* are all as unique as you are. As you read the journeys and experiences of the women in this book, I hope you find inspiration and a spark that leads you to discover or *rediscover* the power in your *sensuality*.

'Don't ask for permission to do, be or receive!
Set your world in motion and create the life you want!'

- Carrie Myers

Pacing Behind the Gate
by Carrie Myers

Are you caged? Pacing back-and-forth, waiting on someone to leave the gate open? Do you feel a longing, like you are coming out of your skin? Daily, you follow the regimen, but you just want to skew a little to the left and leave the chores undone and no dinner on the table. Are you flat with little emotion or laughter? Is wine your comfort after a long day?

Are you ready to sway, dance, laugh, move, explore, grow, take deeper breaths and howl? As women, we aren't built to be stick straight, ticking off tasks and just accomplishing THINGS! For what, they just get undone and need to get re-done tomorrow. Where is the life in that? Where is the flow, the ease, the beauty, and the *sensuality*? Where is your soul's purpose or your authentic self? Where is your happiness and fulfilment? Where is your joy? Where is your connection?

Step out of your box, your cage – let yourself out to freedom. Don't ask for permission to do, be or receive! Set your world in motion and create the life you want! Take it because it is already yours! You were born to be free, wild, happy! You were born to dance, laugh and move in *sensual*, exotic ways – no matter who is watching.

What is Sensuality?
by Carrie Myers

S ensuality: what does that word mean to you? How does it make you feel to hear or say '*sensuality*'? Does it feel taboo? Does it feel dirty? Or does it feel flowy and exciting? Is this even a word you would use? Can you ever say that you have been sensual or felt sensual? If not, why does sensuality evade you?

Why is it that sensuality is not separate from sexuality? Or is it? So much of what we learn does not separate the two. But they are separate. Not all sex is sensual and not all sensuality is sexual. Why has no one defined them separately before now? I can't explain how it is I feel so adamant about this, but I do. Sensuality is a way of being sexual. But sexuality doesn't always include the sensual. Sometimes sex is carnal or fierce. Sometimes sex is indifferent or impersonal. Sometimes sex is fast and hard.

However, sometimes sensuality wants to take her time.

Sensuality is flowy, gentle, soft, lustful and a vastly different experience than just the act of being sexual.

Sensuality is a movement, a way of being. Sensuality can be experienced in the way you dance, eat, groom, read, speak, write and every other aspect of your life. Sensuality is an ease and trust within yourself, feeling confident and feminine. You can be sensual as you dress or undress. Being sensual also includes being authentic, open, confident, unique, and tender.

Why have the two been lumped together and not seen as separate ways of being?

Let us explore the differences and see where it leads us.

'The inquisitiveness of the human mind, body, heart, and soul is what perpetuates us into growth, discovery, and pleasure.'

- Carrie Myers

CURIOSITY, IMAGINATION AND SENSUALITY

by Carrie Myers

Within this world of vast information flowing toward us at lightning speed endlessly, we do not even have to think anymore. We just sit back and absorb whatever someone puts in front of us, without questioning any of it. I have witnessed the demise of creativity and imagination in our school systems, as my children grew bored and uninspired. Sitting in a restaurant, I notice everyone on their phones and playing games, hunched over that cold piece of metal and glass, not connecting, not talking, and not laughing. I wonder what will become of this world as all the information is in a little box and none in our minds. Will we stop creating new inventions? Will we grow listless and withdrawn from one another? Will the laughter of children on a playground cease to exist as they no longer chase, explore, and build sandcastles and mud pies from the earth? Will new stories fail to be written, no poetry to fill the timeless emotions held within?

There is a deep need for curiosity and imagination in this world. Without it, we are stagnant, bored, lonely, and empty. What if you never reached out to touch a puppy and pet his soft fur or smelled his puppy breath? What if you were never curious as to what chocolate tasted like and never knew the smooth, sweet essence of the melting orgasm in your mouth? What if you never turned on the radio to hear Céline Dion sing 'My Heart Will Go On?' What if you never looked up at the beauty and awe of a full moon on a clear, crisp night? What if the world was 72 degrees all the time and you never felt the warmth of a summer day, sweat trickling down your back or the coziness of a wool blanket and a blazing fire on a cold winter night? What if you never felt a sweet, longing, sensual hand running down your arm?

Without curiosity, would our senses become numb, and our life be, well, lifeless?

The inquisitiveness of the human mind, body, heart, and soul is what perpetuates us into growth, discovery, and pleasure.

As we seek out the renewal of sensuality, we cannot forget to infuse curiosity and imagination into our being. Deep in our sacral chakra lies our curiosity, creativity, imagination, sexuality, and sensuality. Society has muted this part of our being with all the shoulds, rules, and boxes that we must check off during our lives. Especially as women, we are shamed for exploring this part of our bodies and minds. Letting go of the expectations of society and getting in touch with our curiosity and creativity can open us back up to the childlike awe that we long to connect with once again.

How can we begin to reconnect with this part of ourselves?

Meditation can ignite the flames of sensuality within us. Close your eyes and send you attention to the sacral chakra, just below your belly button and above your pelvic floor. Envision a spiral of orange energy stirring up the sediment in your pelvis. Allow the swirls to excavate the gunk that has clogged up your sensuality and creative flow. As you exhale, release the sediment into the air. Continue this meditation for 5-10 minutes, returning to it often as you need.

Grounding and play are essential to get in touch with your curiosity and your body. Walk or stand barefoot in the grass. Take walks in the woods to get back in touch with nature. Play in a mud puddle and dance in the rain. Swing until the height grabs your tummy and you giggle. Finger paint with your best friend. You get the idea... Play! And then to deepen the sensual and sexual connection, take play into the bedroom.

Journaling your thoughts and dreams, writing poetry and drawing can shine light on the places that are blocked or renewed. As you write about what you discover about yourself, it gives validity and accountability to your thoughts and authenticity. Record what you feel from every sense and every environment. Bringing these perceptions to life will give you a more tangible sensations and appreciation to your journey and your body.

Create a community with other sensuality seekers. As women come together and open to our needs, desires and quests for connection and sensuality, we discover that we are not alone in our stagnation and desire for more sensuality in our lives. Collaborating on renewal of our feminine energy shifts our lives and ultimately the world to be a gentler, more compassionate, and flowing place.

Read. Read other women's experiences with their discovery of self and rediscovery of their sensual side. Read erotica, romance, spiritual books, and anything else that piques your interest. I recently reread *Are You There God? It's Me, Margaret* by Judy Blume. Talk about taking me back to a time of innocence and curiosity... This book refreshed my girly sense of wonder about my body and my femininity. I highly recommend reading a book that you found intriguing in the fifth grade.

Have gratitude. Sometimes expressing gratitude is the hardest hurdle. But reframing our struggles by looking at our growth and the lessons we have learned is the greatest gift. Gratitude puts our journey into perspective and allows us to see ourselves in a different light. Simple gratitude for your health, your awareness and your renewed curiosity can be enough to set you on the right path to the rediscovery of all you are meant to be in this world.

So where are you going to begin in the journey to reigniting your curiosity, your awe, your sense of self and your sensuality?

Well congratulations, you are already on your way, just by picking up this book. You are about to bear witness to the journey of several women who began asking questions, breaking free from their cages, grabbed their sensuality by the sacral chakra and dove deep within themselves to shine from their sensual souls.

Grab my hand, sister, and let's rummage through the sediment to reclaim our very sensual selves.

""Here you are," the river whispered, holding me safe, holding me brave. "Here you are, I have been waiting for you.""
- Annette Vaucanson Kelly

SKINNY DIP
by Annette Vaucanson Kelly

Swim Nude & Free

In blistering heat, we – all six of us – trekked through the seared silent trees, down a gravelly trail hewn by stormwaters, leading to a shadeless gorge of sun-baked limestone crags and terraces. The rugged flagstones and porous slabs, carved by the oft temperamental Ardèche River and strewn here and there with a few green tufts, bore the scars of many a raging flood. Wave after rowdy wave of brightly coloured canoes drifted down the placid, midnight blue river, and countless holidaymakers and sunbathers already lined its banks. Yet I couldn't shake off the feeling that we were not supposed to be there. Three months of Covid lockdowns and social distancing had utterly frazzled my understanding of how to move in the world.

All afternoon, we swam and jumped and dove into the balmy river. As the crowds made their way up and out of the gorge back to their cars and the flow of canoes down the river trickled out, we unhastily started packing up.

I retrieved a stray pair of goggles from beneath a damp towel. 'I think I'd like to go for one last dip', I confessed to B in a hushed voice. 'Just one more', I added, 'topless.' That last word hung for a second over the orange microfibre towel he was folding. But he simply shrugged his shoulders and smiled a can't-see-why-not kind of smile.

I walked back to the stone step we had used all afternoon and looked all around. One man was watching his son jump in from the high rocks of the opposite bank. At long last, and after much faffing, they finally made to leave. Alone at last.

The sun still crested the limestone cliffs and crags around us, but the gorge was now bathed in welcome shade. At the edge of the river, I slid into the cool dark water and furtively took off my bikini top. I glanced up at B; he met my gaze with a reassuring look and a cheeky grin. I kicked off, swimming breaststroke upstream.

The flutters of my racing heart soon calmed down, all self-consciousness quenched by an unspoken desire to swim unbridled – literally, "not fitted with a bridle". And it felt deliciously bold and subversive.

I soon swam back to shore and, without climbing out of the water, wriggled out of my bikini bottoms, which I flung on the rock beside my abandoned bra.

Back into the depths I went. With a deep exhale I surrendered to the moment. Shackles came off that I didn't realise were there before. *'Here you are,'* the river whispered, holding me safe, holding me brave. *'Here you are. I have been waiting for you, beloved.'*

Slowly I swam downstream towards a bend in the river that was still ablaze with sunlight. Alone in the gentle flow I swam, treaded water, floated on my back. Free. The river welcomed me in her deep embrace, held me in her cool caress. Her fluent touch on my bare breasts and between my legs felt like nothing I had experienced before – intensely sensual but not sexual. Bliss.

In an early scene of French film *Manon des Sources*, Manon "of the springs", unaware she is being watched, hums light-heartedly as she gets undressed in a wildflower meadow by a clear babbling stream. Her long blond hair swishes through the sunny air as she dances to her own tune, and wades naked into the cool crystalline water.

Manon des Sources is a young woman raised in the fragrant hills of Provence by a crone. Wishing to avenge her father's death, caused by local farmers who got hold of his land, she secretly cuts off the village's water supply. *"La sauvageonne"*, the villagers call her, with a mixture of fear and lust.

I was in my mid-teens when I first saw the film on TV. My childhood best friend, raised a good Catholic girl like me, thought the skinny dip scene "quite unnecessary". I found it beautiful. It stirred in me a yearning I couldn't put into words. I longed for Manon's intimate knowledge of the land that raised her. But most of all, I craved her wildness, alluring and troubling.

'Couvrez ce sein que je ne saurais voir', religious zealot Tartuffe instructs Dorine in Molière's eponymous play – a cornerstone of the post-primary curriculum. *'Couvrez ce sein que je ne saurais voir. Par de pareils objets les âmes sont blessées.'* Cover this bosom that I dare not see, for by such objects the soul is tainted.

One time, it must have been before Easter, during an assembly in the school chapel, the parish priest informed us that the sacrament of confession was available to those who wished to repent. To his audience of noisy teenagers, bored witless but still glad for the break from regular classes, he loudly insisted on the need to confess any impure thoughts or deeds.

I squirmed.

Sitting on a wooden pew among peers who didn't give a toss, stewing in my winter coat in the packed chapel, it was as if the priest was talking directly to me. As a child, I had struggled to come up with bagatelles to confess, but this time, I knew exactly, uncomfortably, excruciatingly, what the priest was after. I was *guilty*. Guilty of pleasuring myself, late at night, under the covers of my bed. I longed to relieve my conscience. But in the end, I kept my shame to myself, instead of handing it over to the old man behind the wooden screen to peck at.

I grew up in a Catholic household in rural France that didn't place much value on looks or physical appearance. Yet at the same time, there was this paternalistic assumption that being a girl was a burden, an unlucky dip, a flaw to overcome, through hard work and self-abnegation. Women were not the fairer sex, but the weaker sex.

'*Mon Dieu, je vous l'offre,*' my granny used to mutter as she scrubbed the floors of the local tax office, to earn a pittance that would help pay the rent and feed her four children. She lived through the war alone with her first child, while waiting for the uncertain return of my grandad, taken as a prisoner of war in 1940. She knew to not want too much, to be grateful for what she had.

Like my grandmother, like all women, I learned to distrust my desire, to not want too much. I was made to feel that desire is dirty, selfish, a weakness. To succumb to one's desire is to fail.

I didn't learn to swim as a child. Or rather, I was never taught. My parents, themselves non-swimmers, had a healthy wariness of water and didn't regard swimming as a valuable life skill. So my first time in the local pool was with my class, aged 7. I looked enviously at two of the boys who could already swim – the front crawl, of course. A coach taught the full class the very basics and put us through some drills. But mostly, we were left to our own devices. And it was fun.

I stopped enjoying the school swimming sessions when testing was introduced, in secondary school. My sloppy self-taught breaststroke and lack of fitness meant I could hardly complete one length, let alone 10 laps. On a marking scale set at national level for each year group, I didn't make the bottom rung, scoring a humiliating 5 percent "for good effort".

A few years later, while on an end-of-year school trip, I nearly drowned in the wave pool of a waterpark. The artificial waves relentlessly pulled me past the safe point, towards the wall, closer still, going over my head, until I slipped under, silently. When the lifeguard caught me, I dug my nails into his shoulder and pushed him away, thinking he was a friend holding me under "as a joke", the way teenagers do. He carried me back to safety, back to my friends, and left after checking I was OK. I never saw his face. Shaken, still shaking, and mortified, I asked my friends to keep mum. My near drowning was never spoken of again.

My body was a liability – always too clumsy, too hairy, too inadequate. I was embarrassed by it, this female body which always had the potential to attract unwanted attention, yet not good enough to seduce the boys I fancied, not fit enough to shine in PE lessons, not strong enough to fend off violence. It was like travelling in a leaky hot air balloon – something too soft, too cumbersome, too fickle, to ever feel truly safe in. At any given time, it could betray me – me and my desperate hunger.

Good girls don't want.

What, then, about the simmering dragon in my centre, ravenous, flaring its fiery nostrils and flicking its scaly tail? What if it made me disobey, put myself first, and take up space in the world?

Good girls don't want.

Full stop.

Manon des Sources eventually entered polite society when she married the schoolteacher. Having exposed her father's killers in a thrilling plot twist, *"la sauvageonne"* becomes a respectable wife and mother. Once her wildness had served its purpose, it could not be allowed to flourish unchecked anymore.

I always felt inexplicably sad about this happy ending. Now I know why. Patriarchy had claimed her – hide this power that I dare not see, for by such sights the soul is tainted.

One Christmas several years ago, B handed me a plain envelope. It contained a voucher for 4 private swimming lessons at our local pool in Greystones. I received it with a mixture of gratitude and apprehension. One cold grey January morning three weeks later, I turned up at the leisure centre for my first lesson. After checking in at reception, I nervously made my way in the hot and humid pool area, trying to not embarrass myself while looking for the female changing rooms.

I had never been there before. B sometimes took the kids out for a family swim at the weekend, but I would stay home with our youngest, happy to get a couple of hours to myself instead of pretending to have fun in a setting that felt alien. I have never been the mum to play with our children much. The first years of my love story with B had awakened a playful, sensual me I didn't know I was. But a traumatic first birth experience had left me reeling, seemingly betrayed by my body once more ("failure to progress" is what it reads on my labour notes), and I fell back into my serious ways. I stopped being "selfish" to aim for selfless instead – the gold standard of motherhood.

That first lesson went by in the wink of an eye. Self-consciousness meant that I never fully relaxed into it, but the instructor's gentle manner and good-humoured patience got me through. I only ever had four swimming lessons with him. Nevertheless, once a week after the morning school run, I would drive to the leisure centre for a swim. Every so often, the instructor would be there, either on lifeguard duty or coaching somebody else. And he would kindly offer tips and advice that were crucial to my progress.

It was weeks before I completed a full length without stopping, months before I could swim five laps in under an hour, and even longer until I felt I had earned the right to swim in a lane – the slow lane, of course! I invested in a swimsuit and a new microfibre towel. Swimming became a weekly affair, something I did for myself, by myself. Then, five months after that initial lesson, I took my first dip in the Irish Sea.

In *Waterlog*, Roger Deakin writes, *'Walking, cycling and swimming will always be subversive activities'* because *'they allow us to regain a sense of what is old and wild by breaking free of the official version of things.'*

With my first skinny dip, I swam free of the authorised version of myself. Reclaiming my body as me – a fully-formed human being, not a mere sexual object for the world to gawk at and assess my worthiness on, I was witnessed in my naked fullness, not only by B and our children, but by the river herself, the rocks, the dipping sunlight and the cool shade. Shedding shame like layers of clothing, I was seen as I am. Naked, vulnerable and wild. Sinful and self-full.

This is me. Unashamedly.

Succumb

In this bruising world of guilty pleasure,
Seek the sensual embrace of a skinny dip;
Savour the soft caress of sea on skin.
Succumb to the sweet juicy ápple of knowing
   and become succulent
   and dance.

Surrender to the soul song of the sea
   calling you home to yourself.

The opposite of crying is not laughter,
   it is to sing.
So sing. Scream if need be.
If to be is to sin,
   Sin big
   Bigger still,
Your desire true to the stars that spell it.

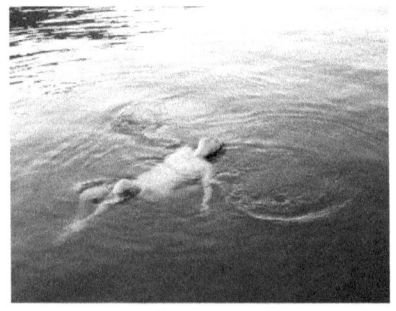

About Annette Vaucanson Kelly

Annette Vaucanson Kelly is a writer, mother and wild swimmer. A former blogger and climate activist, she writes about nature, feminism and mothering, to heal the story of who we are on this achingly beautiful planet. She is French and lives by the Irish Sea in Greystones, Co. Wicklow, Ireland, with her Irish husband and their four children.

Find her on Substack at *Another World is Possible* – https://substack.com/@annettevaucansonkelly

*"You are not lost, my darling,
we are just here to help you remember."*
- Katie May's Soul Guides

Remembering My Sensual, Soulful Self
by Katie May

When I was a little girl I always loved wearing dresses. It made me feel so flowy and free. My body felt free to breathe. When I started kindergarten, one of my first memories of having my sensuality dulled was being asked to wear shorts under my dress. I was livid and I didn't really understand. This was the first of many experiences I would go through where I felt my sensuality being asked to hide.

For many years a journey of disconnection from my body and sensual expression unraveled. Growing up in a conservative, purity culture also added layers of shame and complexity to understanding my thoughts, feelings, needs, wants, and desires. The messages I received were *'ladies keep their legs crossed, wear panty hose, and don't show too much skin.'* As I got older, the messages elevated into *'good girls don't have sex outside of marriage and definitely don't sleep around'*, and *'what you wear might make a man stumble.'* I even had some sexual experiences that seemed to validate some of these messages, so I became even more confused and convinced that my sensuality must be bad.

Naturally, when sensuality turned into sexuality as I got older, I was living in shame and fear of my own body – her sensation, pleasure, and turn on were censored due to the deep shame I felt. I shut it all down, including my creative spirit, and instead went on a conventional path of all the things I thought I "should" do. I went to college, got a degree, and when I did marry at the ripe age of 22 it was all supposed to just magically turn back on and be OK, right?

It didn't.

It took 12 years of marriage, coming into motherhood, and the unraveling and rebuilding of that marriage after the news of an affair in the first 2 years of it that really sent me on a wild journey of sensual and sexual reclamation. I let the anger, rage, betrayal, love, grace, forgiveness, and finally peace surge through me over and over again until I felt I could move forward. My first steps were waking back up to my own body, her wisdom, and to learning how to allow pleasure and connection to my own sensual soul and self.

I am still on this journey, this path of sensual and sexual awakening and remembrance. Now, as a mother of two amazing daughters, I realize my greatest responsibility is not only to myself and my own inner child, but also to freeing them from having to carry any further shame, disconnection, or fear around sensuality from generations of women who were oppressed and not allowed to live from their own sensual soul. We are the cycle breakers, healing for ourselves and also healing our lineage past, present, and future.

We get to write a new story of our sensual experience on this earth.

We get to liberate our bodies and our souls as we remember the medicine our sensual nature brings to this earth.

It is healing.

We are healing.

Sensual Mama

Her motherhood journey awakens her.

Teaches her things nothing else could.

Connecting her to a deeper sense of...

life

creatrix

source

the Goddess

She rises in love and also holds her own shadow.

She knows the secret to the Magic is in her own window.

Her soul is deep and unapologetic about its musings.

The medicine, here for our using.

Lessons, upon lessons infuse her.

Every cell awakening to the divine love within.

She is made of love and therefore cannot truly sin.

For she knows it's all part of her humanness, to give and receive.

When she is plugged in to her highest self, true peace she can achieve.

Her sensual, sexual flow knows the way.

A healer in her own way, here to hold the space for humanity.

Mothering all and mothering her.

She is ready to embrace the call.

She flows with love and grace for all.

Her heart has been expanded and it shows.
She has connected herself back to herself
It's easy to know...
The softness of her body
The flow of her desire
A life giver and nurturer, she does not tire
She owns her energy from a place of abundance, not scarcity
She has fire and tenacity
A woman unto herself
Sovereign, divine, and holy
Pleasure filled and over flowing
Turned on by life
Her authenticity showing
She knows no limits
She is guided and loved
Held with a sacred energy from above.

About Katie May

Katie May is a Sacred Feminine and Soul Embodiment Coach who believes in the power of women and their bodies.

She is an avid lover of connection and creating safe and sacred spaces for women to own their magic and tap into their own wildly sacred life through seasonal and cyclical living. She helps you get back in your body, reconnect to your inner wisdom, and lead from your soul.

Her offerings weave through Akashic Frequency and Heart, Wild Mother Love, and Sacred Feminine Wisdom.

With over 15 years of experience as a nurse in palliative and end of life care, she has learned so much about the resilience of the human spirit and also a deep desire for all of us to be seen, heard, and known. She practices in a way that honors the story of each individual and helps to elicit the deeper connection to the healing within.

Katie is a native of the Mountains of NC where she resides today with her partner of 18 years, two daughters, and healing pup Wilder.

> You can connect with Katie through her
> Instagram @embraceyourselfwhole

'My journey of reclaiming myself as
a good and sexy Vietnamese woman had to
start off with first liberating myself to
the concept that I could be both.'
- Elizabeth Nguyen

The Good and Sexy Vietnamese Woman
by Elizabeth Nguyen

My mother and I didn't talk about sex growing up. We didn't talk about sex when I became a young woman, or when I got married, or when I got divorced. I'm pretty sure most Vietnamese women of my mother's generation don't talk to their daughters about sex. The sex education I received from my parents was unspoken and unseen. That was how we were taught to relate to sex: unspoken and unseen. In fact, I still don't know how to say the word "sex" in Vietnamese, even though it was my parents' native language that was spoken to me throughout my childhood. As good Vietnamese daughters and wives, my sisters and I were taught to tend to our husbands and children as the highest priority. There was no mention of how we got pregnant, what sexual desire was, or whether sex was even an important part of a woman's life.

Whether it was explicitly explained to me or not, I learned that *good* Vietnamese women were wives and mothers who took care of their families. *Sexy* Vietnamese women, on the other hand, were party girls who were irresponsible and drank too much. Good Vietnamese women always put their children's needs ahead of their own. Sexy Vietnamese women were indecent and selfish. Good Vietnamese women dressed a certain way that communicated their propriety and respectability. Sexy Vietnamese women displayed too much of their skin and were immoral with their exposure and behaviors. It seemed impossible to be *both* a good Vietnamese woman and a sexy Vietnamese woman.

This education I received about the difference between a good Vietnamese woman and a sexy Vietnamese woman was very confusing, because even as they weren't favorably judged, sexy Vietnamese women commanded a lot of attention and space in the Vietnamese psyche. While simultaneously being disapproved of, sexy Vietnamese women were turning a lot of heads. I recall attending Vietnamese parties with my parents and their friends and hearing the adults endlessly notice and compare every woman in the room for her looks, and comment on her hair, makeup, and what she was wearing. They noticed the women who were sexy. But if she was dressed *too* sexy (and everyone had their own opinion about what too sexy was) she would be judged as inappropriate. It was hard to know what *too* sexy was.

The traditional Vietnamese dress known as the áo dài is the epitome of the conflicting messages Vietnamese girls and women have been taught about our beauty and sexuality. The áo dài is an article of clothing "that covers everything, but hides nothing." The áo dài is overtly designed to covertly display the sensual feminine beauty of the Vietnamese woman. Even though its traditional high-collared neck, long sleeves, and floor-length silk pants cover a Vietnamese woman from head to toe, its form-fitting cut closely hugs every contour of the female form, as if it is touching and caressing her body the way she wants to be touched and caressed. The well-placed slits along the side seams of the áo dài are carefully measured to end just above the waistline of the silk pants, to purposely reveal a glimpse of a woman's bare skin when she and her dress move a certain way in the wind. The áo dài seems to tell young Vietnamese girls: *you are beautiful, people like to admire your beauty, and we want you to be a symbol for the beauty of our culture and people*. But at the same time it also tells young Vietnamese girls: *you can't be too sexy, you have to cover yourself up, you can't show your body to others, that can be dangerous*. These opposing messages leave a very narrow tightrope for a Vietnamese girl to traverse as she makes her way from adolescence to young adulthood. Sometimes it feels like too narrow a path to walk, and it's just easier to fall to either side. On one side – *don't bring attention to yourself, hide your looks, hide your sexuality, and focus on other things besides your appearance.* The other side – *wear your sexuality and sensuality openly, don't censor it or cover it up, and in fact, work it, it's what people want and expect from you.*

As a gangly young teenager with a developing body, I had no idea how to navigate this complex terrain of my physical appearance and sexuality in just the right way that it honored me, and respected my family and my culture. That's a tall task for an adolescent. So I chose the option of just ignoring the task.

I paid very little attention to my physical appearance and sexuality as a Vietnamese girl and young woman for a long time. I was always naturally more of a tomboy growing up anyway, preferring to wear shorts and T-shirts that made physical activity and sports easier. When I had to choose something to wear, I usually chose comfort over appearance. I purposely wore modest clothing that wouldn't bring much attention to my body or my looks. I dreaded events and occasions where I was expected to dress up because I didn't really know how to do it, and I always felt uncomfortable with it. Of course, there were moments and times where I was aware that I "cleaned up nice" or that I had the ability to "look pretty," but I doubted my own physical attractiveness as a girl and woman well into my late thirties. I grew up with two older sisters who were much more knowledgeable and skilled than I was in all those things that I dubbed "feminine" – hair, makeup, clothing, shoes, accessories, posing for photos, etc. I was the smart one, the tomboy, the bookworm. I hid behind those identities and well-covered comfortable clothes because, well, it was just more comfortable there.

My 40th birthday party that I threw for myself to celebrate my sensual self was the first time I felt comfortable putting on a sexy red dress, and wearing Ferrari-red lipstick that I didn't dab away to "tone it down." Red had always been too much of an attention-getting color for me, but now I understood it – people wear red to grab other people's attention. It wasn't until I felt comfortable seeing myself as a sexy, attractive woman that I could feel comfortable being seen by others that way as well.

My journey of reclaiming myself as a good and sexy Vietnamese woman had to start off with first liberating myself to the concept that I could be both. I didn't have to choose one or the other, and being one didn't preclude being the other. Since I had chosen to be a good Vietnamese woman for most of my life instead of a sexy one, discovering my sexy identity became somewhat of a treasure hunt for something that had been deeply buried. I was initially as shy as the adolescent schoolgirl who was originally faced with this task and had turned the other way. But before turning away, I recalled that my young adolescent self had always felt a strong sexual energy. My sexual self had always been there with me from the beginning. I remembered becoming aroused when I watched soap operas with my older sisters, or when I looked at pictures of attractive couples making out in Cosmo magazine. I touched myself and rubbed myself against a pillow until I orgasmed. I fantasized about kissing and having sex. But at some point, I put this side of myself away. I stored her away in a precious lacquered box until she was ready for me to come and find her again.

For many years, I pushed my sexuality underground in service to my education, my children, and my career. I felt her bubbling underneath the surface, but I was too busy being the good girl, the good doctor, the good wife, and the good mother to give my sexual self much time to explore herself. But as someone committed to deeply knowing myself, my journey inevitably led me back to my sexuality. I couldn't run away from my sexuality anymore. She was the vast source of so much of who I was, and who I was becoming. When I did finally return to reclaim her, I wanted to undress the layers of my sexuality not because anyone else told me I should, or because I had to, but because I *wanted* to. I wanted to know my sexual self underneath everything I had been taught by my family, my culture, my peers, by society, and by the media. All of that had influenced the development of my sexuality, but it was from an external source. I wanted to discover and experience my sexuality from the inside out. What does my body want? What is my body curious about? What turns me on? What turns me off? What makes my body feel good? How do I feel when I am inhabiting my sensual sexual self and how does this interact with my partner's sexuality? Who do I see when I look at myself in the mirror and admire my sexy, sensual self? What is she wearing? How is she holding herself? How is she moving her body? How does it feel to truly let go and surrender?

All of these questions and answers took time for me to explore and experience. I became my own lover, and explored my body in the way she wanted to be explored, both by myself and with my partner. I am still exploring and experiencing. Like any terrain, there is infinite depth and expanse to be uncovered. My sexuality was waiting for me in that precious box to come back and find her after all those years, and as I rediscovered her, I also had to face that there was a loss. A loss of time, of experience, of my sexual youth. I needed to grieve this loss as part of my journey. It also took time for me to peel back the layers of shame and shyness around my sexuality in order for her to come out more fully. Was it really OK for me as a good Vietnamese woman to also be a sexual Vietnamese woman? My Vietnamese identity and culture will always play a part in my sexuality. Even as I am openly writing this essay about my sexuality, I know that my sexuality also is very private to me, its intimate details only to be shared in safe and trusted spaces.

But one thing I now know for certain is that my sexuality is very important to me. I have a strong sex drive. I love having sex. I love both the emotional intimacy of the act and the physical sensations of it. I love how it is the most sacred and intimate way I can connect with myself and my partner. I love how my body feels engaging in the entire sexual space from desire to arousal to playing in the erotic space to connecting deeply with my partner with trust, love, surrender, and abandon. Expressing my sexual self is important to me feeling whole, seen, felt, and desired. My sexual self is a big part of who I am. She inhabits me every moment of my life, not just in the bedroom.

As I raise my own Vietnamese-Mexican-American daughter, I want her to know that sex is a natural and important part of a woman's life. I want her to know that her sexuality is a beautiful, sacred, and powerful part of her identity that deserves as much time and attention to nurturing and developing as any other part of her identity.

I want her to know that she can talk to me about sex. I want her to know that good and sexy sex is a meaningful and pleasurable part of her life and a healthy relationship. I want her to know that she can be a *good and sexy* Vietnamese-Mexican-American woman.

About Elizabeth Nguyen

Elizabeth Nguyen, MD is a Vietnamese-American writer and psychiatrist. She was born and raised in Honolulu, Hawaii. Her parents were refugees from Vietnam who arrived in Honolulu in 1975 at the end of the Vietnam War. She received her BA from Stanford University in Human Biology, her MD from Northwestern University, and her Psychiatry Residency and Child Psychiatry Fellowship training at UC Davis. She started her career in community mental health, with specific interests in cross-cultural psychiatry, the intersection of spirituality and mental health, and the healing power of water and the natural world. What makes her sensual soul shine are playing in water and the beauty of the natural world, sex, hot springs, yoga, massage, dancing, vibrant food, connection, and depth. She currently lives and works in private practice in Davis, CA.

You can find her at
www.multidimensional.psychiatry.com.

'She's taking it all in as she flows with the land.'

- Carrie Myers

The Masculine and Feminine Take a Hike

by Carrie Myers

He laces up his shoes and grabs his water bottle
He says *'let's go'*
She pulls her hair up
Grabs her favorite gemstones
Decorates her body with necklaces and earrings
and finally, she is ready
They arrive at the foot of the trail
His goal – to make it to the top as quick as possible
Her goal – to enjoy the day and see where it takes her
He heads up the trail thinking she's right behind
He huffs and puffs, getting his heart rate high
Never looking up until he's at the peak
He looks around and she is nowhere to be found
Where is she?
Meanwhile, she's making her way, slowly
She is taking pictures, picking flowers,
Talking to the birds and squirrels
Her shoes are in her hand, her feet are in the stream
She's taking it all in as she flows with the land
Will she make it to the top?
Absolutely –
Just not in a hard, straight line and all in due time

Take a few minutes to sit in nature and just feel the love of the earth and Mother. Journal what comes up for you and how you feel after honoring nature.

RECLAIM YOUR SENSUALITY WITH NATURE

by Carrie Myers

I do believe that part of reclaiming *sensuality* is getting back in touch with nature. Think about how Mother Nature does not follow the straight and narrow. She cries rain when she is sad, and storms when she is angry – allowing her emotions to flow. Her trees and plants are resilient and strong, pushing their way through the dirt to bloom in the sun, using the rain as it comes. Trees grow around obstacles and stones and never straight up like an arrow (the masculine). They sway in the breeze and flow, leaves turning and holding on in the wind. Nothing is perfect, but still, it is immaculate in nature. Nature is also not competitive, as it allows space for all and even creates beds for the rivers and streams. Holding the water with a strong hug of the banks, it allows the flow to be gentle, yet determined. The rocks allow the water to fall over them as they acquiesce to the purity of the water as they shine through. Waterfalls emit the beat to keep us in harmony with Mother's rhythm. The wildlife seeks balance and never takes more than they need. Insects clean up all that is left in decay and death – once again reaching for that gentle balance that is ever so delicate. The earth, dirt, and ground holds us and heals us with her love.

So, flow like a river. Dance like a tree. Bloom like a flower. Nurture yourself like the earth. Take what you need and desire, but nothing more. And shine like the sun.

'What would the flow of femininity feel like as it infiltrated the world?'

- Carrie Myers

FINDING SENSUALITY IN THE MASCULINE WORLD

by Carrie Myers

I believe sensuality is elusive to many women. In a society that values the strong masculine, which is all about doing, logic, action, strength, power, and efficiency, it has begun to drown out the feminine side of societies around the globe. The feminine – full of empathy, nurturing, fluidity, openness, creativity, intuition, and compassion – has all but evaporated in the patriarchal, get it done, non-stop world. Women, striving to be competitive with the iron suits and high salaries of large companies, put aside their natural flow to stand up to the survival of the fittest in the masculine world.

Now, I am not saying that women do not belong in the corporate world, because we all know that is just not true. Women can do anything they set their minds to. What I am saying, is that we have put aside the exquisite powers and energies of the feminine to live in and compete in the masculine driven society, in the masculine way. And this makes our world out of balance. What would the divine feminine bring to the masculine corporate world?

Can you see it?

Our earth is overwhelmed with war, pride, narcissism, hunger for power, success, money, and control driven mentalities. Most of this being the shadow side of the masculine. As women, we have been forced to suppress our nurturing, intuition-driven, soft, and empathetic nature to prove our worth and strength in the *man's world.*

So much masculine energy seeps into our feminine and drowns her under his strong arm.

Most women I speak to feel lost in their sensuality, sexuality, desires, needs and purpose. Most are not even sure what sensuality means or what they want? Most feel stagnant and exhausted in their routines and chores.

Isn't it time to regain our nature, our soft side, our receptive side, our pleasure, and our flow?

Sensuality is so much more than sex, even though sensuality can be intertwined with your sexuality.

What if confidence within your sensuality allows for a deeper sexual connection with your partner? What if sensuality was met with curiosity and depth? What if we see sensuality as movement, flow, gentleness, empathy, and confidence in the way a woman carries herself? What if women embody the divine femininity through every breath, movement, conversation and the care for ourselves and others?

'All that remains after a transformation process like this is the truest, most innocent, purest version of you – left to walk this human existence and show there is another way – the sensual way where every moment has the potential to light every cell of your body and soul on fire with the energy of pleasure, peace, joy and unconditional love. Even the moments of deep grief can become this, if the sensual channels are open, because the frequency of this pain is alchemized into and by unconditional love. It is here where all is embraced and given equal space to be felt and experienced. This is living life wide open and ready to experience it in its fullest, one sensual moment at a time.'

– Heather Robbins

LIVING LIFE WIDE OPEN
by Heather Robbins

Sensuality = nourishing my body, heart, mind and soul... in whatever way, shape or form the current moment is calling for

It was with my husband's passing that the reality I had been living in shattered and every piece of me and who I knew myself to be imploded, exploded and crumbled all at once. It was in this raw energy of utter death that I was purified; as my reality began to transform it began asking me to purify and alchemize all that once was. In these fires of transformation I was held by the Mother/Father God within and my heart and every cell of my being was opened to unconditional love. Here, Spirit walked me through the Bardo State and I was shown all the ways in which I did not love myself, my husband and many countless others in my life well. This came in flashes of moments from the past where I thought I had acted from love, but really it was my fear or conditioning or epigenetic tendencies that caused me to act the way I did. I was shown how far we, as a society, have strayed from operating from a place of love and instead operate out of fear and how we have settled for this and have come to believe it to be love. It is in these moments, these flashes, where the pain of how I wished things had been different was ultimately shown to me to all be for the spiritual and soul growth of everyone involved. This is when unconditional love would come pouring in and hold me as I cried. As grace and compassion held me and the fires burned and purified all that was not love, I began to feel my energy body, spiritual body, and emotional body come back online and lighten.

I spent a couple months walking the Bardo State and it was during this time my Kundalini was activated. It was a powerful energy that shot from my root chakra up my spine and ignited my spiritual and physical vessel so that every cell, every chakra, literally every inch of me was lit up. In the days and weeks and months that followed I opened myself more and more to the spiritual journey of inner union, personal alchemy, and full circle transformation I was being asked to walk. As I walked this path where every moment brought more purification, more edges to move beyond, more and more growth points and choice points for expansion, I began to see how I had lived my life up until my husband's passing filled with fear, and how that had kept my energy from flowing. The fear from my mental body would cause me to doubt myself. This would stagnate decisions and create dissonance and pain in my physical body. My fear of feeling anything that my mind and body perceived as uncomfortable blocked my ability to feel pleasure because as I closed myself off from not only the "bad" in life, I also closed myself off from the "good". I was shown how complex this was as I moved through the explosion of my Kundalini because my sexual, creative energy was very much caught up in belief systems that this energy was "bad" and thoughts that "I am not creative". It was nearly impossible for me to experience my vital energy, my life force, my creative power, my sensuality, on any level because of these belief systems and thought patterns. It is these belief systems and thought patterns of fear that kept me feeling this sense of lack.

Essentially I had no energy to run off of nor do anything with; I felt I couldn't create anything, and I certainly didn't know how to experience anything from a place a joy or pleasure. This way of living kept the very essence of me, Heather, as a being in human form, not only from experiencing life, but it kept me from co-creating WITH life as well. At a certain point everything within me became so overwhelming that I gave into the pain and gave myself permission to feel the mental and emotional discomfort of the situation and circumstances I found myself in and was experiencing. This is where I faced my deepest fears of walking this life alone, being alone, feeling alone, having to make decisions for myself and my children that only I was responsible for and there was no one else there to blame if things went bad or wrong. It was at this time where I began to walk in the Light, my light, again.

This journey began to show me how I had created the reality I had been living in from a place of fear, from the shadows; without heart, without love, without peace in my body, heart, mind and soul. It was through this purification that all these aspects of myself were made known and became clear; I could see how I had not really been living from my truest self. Feeling connected back to my soul and my heart and with clarity in my mind and womb from the purification process, I could see how the soil for my new life was also purified and the seeds for this next chapter were watered and nurtured by my inner Divine Masculine and inner Divine Feminine. It is through this process that I began to feel safe in my body so that I could witness all the deep emotions life was bringing up in me. My ability to allow myself to be and to hold myself kept my channel open and clear, my energy moving so life was then free to create through me.

Feeling, now, how free my energy moves and how freely I follow it reminds me of how free children are when they play. Coming home to myself through this death and rebirth/transformation/purification process has helped me reclaim my innocence for all things pleasurable within my body and with the experiences that come to me each and every day. I can now sit and take myself on a date by going to get a cherry and cream cheese Danish from a pastry shop in town and almost orgasm from the love I feel on every level from myself and the Universe around me. In every moment now I invite love in. I invite it in by calling my attention and focus to the present moment and who I am with through my senses like my touch or my sight. I invite love in when I ask how I can honor my soul in any given moment. And when I invite love in, I open myself in my heart and in my body so that I may receive it fully in whatever shape or form it comes.

Sometimes the unconditional love I feel hurts so badly because it is a love that is so immense it cracks my heart wide open.

To me, all of this, my every experience is the innocence of my soul having this human experience and when it is fully experienced with every sense and every cell and it is embodied, everything can become and then is – sensual. Life is sensual. Life is meant to be experienced unflinchingly and wide open like the Fool who is always ready to experience the next thing no matter what is to come. Life is beautifully, devastatingly, surreally, heartbreakingly, profoundly sensual. It is meant to be stared in the face and breathed in, drank up, and scarfed down at every turn with gusto and gratitude and a "Yes thank you; more please" kind of attitude! Somewhere along the way we became afraid to live so we as a society closed ourselves off, shamed our innocence, guilted each other for too much pleasure, too much fun, too many orgasms and began to normalize living boring, unfulfilled, unmusical, fear-based lives. Before my husband died I was scared all the time. Before my husband died HE was scared all the time. This fear of dying and failing keeps us from living and succeeding. It keeps us in survival mode unable to tap into the very energy that would help us create the lives we truly desire to live. Fear stagnates everything and then we create from a sense of illusion and not the truth of the moment. By facing my ultimate fear all my other fears were brought to the surface to be faced and eventually walked through so that they, too, could be purified from my field.

With all of this I find myself incredibly grateful and powerfully blessed. I feel I have a new lease on life and I owe it to my late husband to live it out and embody what I have learned from our living together and through our dying together. The me that existed before my husband died, died along with him; that girl no longer exists. I have even come to believe she never really existed anyway because she was a shadow of the pure essence I feel I am now and always was; she was an illusion created by the conditioning and programming placed upon her. It is in the moment of facing your fears as I have and walking the fires of purification where everything from before ceases to be. All that remains after a transformation process like this is the truest, most innocent, purest version of you – left to walk this human existence and show there is another way – the sensual way where every moment has the potential to light every cell of your body and soul on fire with the energy of pleasure, peace, joy and unconditional love. Even the moments of deep grief can become this, if the sensual channels are open, because the frequency of this pain is alchemized into and by unconditional love. It is here where all is embraced and given equal space to be felt and experienced. This is living life wide open and ready to experience it in its fullest, one sensual moment at a time.

In love, with gratitude,

Heather

About Heather Robbins

Heather Robbins was born and raised in Zionsville, Indiana. She received her B.A. in Philosophy from Indiana University and went on to receive her Doctorate in Physical Therapy from Miami University. Shortly after beginning work she found herself fascinated by energy medicine and became a HighSpeed Energy Healing™ Practitioner. Her understanding of the physical realm coupled with her passion for energy gives her a unique perspective and ability to facilitate powerful shifts in those she works with. It is her mission to empower souls to align to their natural blueprint so that they may embody their truth in every way. It is her belief that when this is done, a person's inner light can bravely and unapologetically shine for all to see. Heather currently lives in Northern Virginia with her two children.

www.wayshowerwellness.org

'Being truly in my body has been so foreign to me. Something I ran away from with every ounce of my being, especially when feelings felt too much. I now know this is the complete opposite of sensuality. I'm learning how to be present and connect with myself in my body for the first time. Being in my body and out of my mind feels like an out of body experience.'

- Katie Weiper

LOVE NOTES TO ME, FROM THE DEPTHS OF MY SOUL
by Katie Weiper

A pattern I'm working to lose is one of unworthiness, specifically surrounding my career choice. *"I'm just a mom"* my ego has said to me more times than I can count. It makes me incredibly sad that we live in a time where raising our next generation is seen as less than to many. What makes me even more sad? I believed it. I don't have letters after my name. I haven't started a business; I don't have a website and I certainly don't have a following on Instagram. But what I've come to realize is that being "just a mom" is exactly where I'm meant to be because I am living the dream I once had as a child. And yet, somehow society is trying to tell me that I'm not enough. Shouldn't living our dreams be enough? Shouldn't not being a part of the hamster wheel be celebrated? I am seeking out a life where I can deeply connect to myself, nature, my senses, my husband and, most importantly, my children.

I fell into the trap of the masculine world for far too long. Decades of my life were spent people pleasing, completely disconnected from my own feelings, emotions, bodily sensations and needs in order to keep the peace. I now know this is a result of the fawn trauma response but for so much of my life I felt broken. Generation after generation of women in my family were conditioned to stuff our feelings down and put everyone and everything ahead of ourselves. I knew no different and felt this was normal.

To layer on top, I am also a recovering perfectionist. As a need for control from my inner chaos, I learned that attempting to control everything within and around me made me feel "better", more capable and worthy. However, control issues aren't really about lack of control, they stem from a lack of self-trust. For so long, I was told to not trust myself. Because of this, I placed perfectionism expectations on myself and the people around me which took me so far away from being able to experience the present moment. I felt the need to portray perfectionism all as a way to earn love. Because in my old truth, love is earned when I do things perfectly. I thought, *"If I can control being perfect, I can be loved"*. I am breaking free of this conditioning in order to let my true light shine. Perfectionism helped me survive parts of my life where I felt emotionally unsafe. But it no longer serves me. It's not who I am at a soul level. I am ready to live. To love. To experience. To find joy in the mundane and imperfect.

As a result of straying so far away from my intuition and divine purpose, I developed a host of physical and emotional symptoms early on in life that deeply affected my day to day. I experienced my first of many panic attacks as a young girl in elementary school. This was the beginning of debilitating anxiety that ensued daily for decades and influenced my decision to carry Xanax with me at all times to prevent intense panic attacks landing me in the ER. Severe digestive ailments and food intolerances developed as I continued to ignore warning messages my body tried to send me. To top it off, nervous system dysregulation from generational patterns and life traumas which kept me in patterns of flight, fight and freeze made it impossible to connect to my body. Gradually, I got to a place where I felt I couldn't stand up for myself because I no longer knew my truth and always felt the need to constantly make everyone else feel comfortable, making it impossible to advocate for myself. By the time I was 30, I was on 6 daily prescription medications and was seeing a cardiologist for unexplained heart palpitations. All of this medication was a failing Band-Aid as I felt awful physically and emotionally day in and out. I constantly felt like I was missing out on life with my husband and our two young children and knew that wasn't how I wanted to continue living. I knew it was time to approach life from a different lens, to get to the root cause and to begin learning how to listen to and honor my body.

I've hidden many parts of myself out of fear of being rejected, not fully accepted or loved. Eight years into my healing journey that has encompassed all of my 30s, I'm now learning who I am at a soul level and welcoming myself back home each and every day. Being truly in my body has been so foreign to me. Something I ran away from with every ounce of my being, especially when feelings felt too much. I now know this is the complete opposite of sensuality. I'm learning how to be present and connect with myself in my body for the first time. Being in my body and out of my mind feels like an out of body experience. The healing journey isn't easy, but it's certainly worth it. With each new season, I look at things with such wonder. Everything looks clearer and feels new. This journey has made me realize I want to feel this same excitement in my soul each and every day for the rest of my life.

Recently I got the nudge to page through all my journals. I paused what I was doing, collected the most recent ones, and sat down with a cup of tea to begin reading. Journaling has been an important part of my life since I was in middle school. And while my entries certainly look very different now, allowing myself to have a safe space to let my thoughts flow out on to paper has always felt comforting. As I began this process, I was amazed at what I had written. Nothing was carefully thought out ahead of time and yet I felt like so much of what had flowed out on those pages were profound words I need to remind myself of time and time again. I now feel like I'm finally coming home to myself and my truth. I know with each step, I'm getting closer and closer to true embodiment. I feel whole and filled with so much love and joy.

I hope I never forget these love notes that came directly from my soul. I hope that these words will help me to continue to break free of my conditioning and generational patterns. I hope these words serve as a reminder of how beautiful it is to welcome myself home each and every day. I hope these words will continue to encourage me to raise my babies so they never lose sight of who they are, why they are so special and how to connect to their truth no matter what life throws at them. And I dream that these words make their way to women who feel like they are "just a mom", to sweet souls who have been conditioned to feel less than or unworthy, to the fighters that continue their daily battles to uncover the root of their physical and emotional symptoms and any other human needing a boost of love, strength and peace as they continue on this journey that is life.

- Love notes, directly from my soul -

I feel relaxed, at peace and free.

I am not a to-do list.

My worth doesn't live in my production.

I am safe in my body.

I am a bright light to this world.

I open my arms and heart to receive whatever unfolds in my life.

I am releasing the need to know all the answers and am anchored in knowing that we are being supported and guided.

~

Just like the leaves that break free and float away from its tree in the fall, it is okay to break free of who you thought you were. It's okay to break free of the story you've been told that you need to be perfect, quiet and put everyone else first. Let yourself float away to where you're guided. Relinquish control. In order for your dreams to come true, you must stay open to guidance and prepare space for them to unfold in divine timing. Trust that you are on the right path and are being guided back to your essential self. Know that life is unfolding beautifully and perfectly on time. Take risks, live a life full of wonder, exude unconditional love and stand up for what you believe in unapologetically.

~

When I honor myself – thoughts, feelings, sensations, nudges, cues – I grow my capacity of what I can handle and get closer to my soul. The more I ignore, the further away I get from her. Healing has no finish line. There is no prize for how fast I do the work. Growing my capacity in order to live the life I desire, one of truly living and deeply loving, is the goal. Maybe the answers will come when I stop trying so hard. Now is the time to surrender, to listen, to forge forward in my truth and what feels right. I will enjoy life now and know there is so much goodness in this moment. Healing. Freedom. Relaxation. Peace. They are all part of my story.

~

Why have I placed such high expectations on myself to be an expert in me before I actually put in the work? Learning about my truth is like learning a new language. One can't have a conversation fluently in a new language in the first days, weeks or months. It takes time. It takes practice. It takes going back to the basics. When you go back to the beginning of your soul, you can start to understand her. To listen and learn. And that is where true living begins.

~

I am thriving. Tough situations allow me to grow and thrive in life. People seek shelter in my energy and I want to use that as comfort and change. I am strong and I know the best is yet to come. So much goodness surrounds all of us and no matter what, we are being called to make changes that allow us to break free of patterns, rewrite our stories and create a life full of connection, abundance, presence and so much love. Whatever comes, know that ultimately it all is for my highest good.

~

There is so much beauty in the in-between. When it's hot and feels like summer yet the leaves are falling to the ground and goldenrod is in full bloom. When you notice the browning of wildflowers in the field preparing for winter then catch a glimpse of joyous butterflies dancing around searching for the last bit of sweet nectar. The newness of an experience, even as simple as taking a walk in a new location, brings newness to life. Things so simple yet profound that if we don't pay attention, we miss them. For so long, I never knew how much peace and beauty could come in such simplicity. I am noticing now what it feels like to be present and how slowing down allows me to use my senses to bring joy and pleasure to my life. What I'm starting to notice is how often I went throughout the day without thinking, on autopilot. I am learning to find safety within my body, which feels so powerful. I am continually reminded to keep my focus on LIVING and not on healing. Sensuality is the precursor to living. Because one can't truly live without experiencing the world through one's senses. And in doing this, we are able to have more pleasure, in all of life. Connecting to my body and soul through my senses is changing my life. It's shifting my world to one of enjoyment, living, loving and gratitude. The voyage has begun and I'm ready to walk the path back home to myself.

~

You are living the dream you once had. You can either wish it away because it feels different and harder than you imagined. Or you can choose to live and find joy in the pockets of peace and relaxation. Life doesn't need more to-do list items. What it does need more of is stillness and connection to ourselves, nature and each other. We must pair the busy with the boredom. We must pair the productiveness with the peacefulness. Even when life looks and feels different than imagined, continue to stay open, stop trying to control and stop should-ing on yourself. When you do this, you will see how incredible this version of your prayer is that you never could imagine or know could come true. What an incredible responsibility you've been given to raise these four humans. They are your biggest cheerleaders, smartest teachers and largest mirrors challenging you to face your fears, step in to the uncomfortable and live life to the fullest. Your energy is a beautiful, sheltering place for your family to find peace, rest and connection.

~

I am open. I am breaking free and stepping in to my whole truth. I am ready to live a life to my highest potential. I am ready to start anew. For now, I will stay open, grounded, and will release judgment. I know the best is yet to come and I will prepare physically, mentally and emotionally for my deepest desires to unfold. I am so thankful for this journey. For learning how to feel, connect and honor myself. To find peace and love in the life we have created together. To be thankful for all the blessings we have and show grace, not judgment, to others I may not understand. Staying in the comfortable would be easy. But I know that's not where I'm meant to be nor where I'll thrive or be the truest version of myself. My body and soul have been abandoned time and time again and I'm ready to put her first, to honor her, listen to her and regain her trust. I know that I must make room in my heart and life for my desires to manifest. And now I say "yes" to falling in love with me. To love myself and my life so much that I can't stop falling in love with me over and over, in order to then give all my love to the people and things that mean more to me than words could ever describe. Life is so beautiful. When I stop judging myself and drop the expectations, I am able to marvel in all that surrounds me. Giving myself space to feel, grow and heal is what I deserve. I feel like I'm finally coming home to my soul. I feel whole and true and filled with so much love and joy.

About Katie Weiper

Katie Weiper was born and raised in central Indiana. Tapping into her lifelong passion for kids, Katie graduated from Indiana University with a Bachelors in Education. She has a zest for constantly learning and loves teaching and helping others. Spending life with her dream husband whom she met in high school is one of her favorite parts of life. The two live just north of Indianapolis in a suburb with their four beautiful young children and a rambunctious golden retriever, all of whom Katie believes to be her most important teachers. Katie started on a quest to break social constraints, find true health and live authentically and with purpose almost a decade ago. She hopes to encourage those around her to live in their truth and follow their soul's purpose. She will be forever indebted to her late mother-in-law, Lisa, for planting seeds of holistic, true living in Katie's husband and within herself during the time they had together on earth. In her free time, Katie loves reading and learning, being in the sun, especially with her toes in the sand, spending time on the water at their family's lakehouse, snuggled up with her husband and laughing with and learning from her children. Katie enjoys writing and has had a dream of becoming a published author. She is thrilled to be a part of this collaborative book.

'Where I once sought a misguided sexual freedom that disregarded the sanctity of my word and the feelings of others, I'm searching for a sensual, fully embodied, soul-nourishing liberation.'

- Kim Lange (Huynh)

BURNING DOWN THE HOUSE
by Kim Lange (Huynh)

ear Sangha,

We are writing to inform you of the outcome of the investigation into Noah Levine's conduct and the future of Against the Stream Buddhist Meditation Society (ATS). We regret the delay and lengthy period of silence that contributed to uncertainty, confusion and pain..."

My boyfriend and I had been driving on the 80 East for only a few miles, beginning the journey to Black Rock City for our first Burning Man, when the news landed in my inbox. I'd almost forgotten about the investigation, preoccupied by thoughts of the emotional affair that was cut short as abruptly and unexpectedly as it had begun when Adam – who after just a few months and less than a dozen cups of chai teas together had come to mean so much more to me than a friend – packed up his belongings and moved 2,875 miles across the country, intent on giving his faltering relationship one last shot after I'd decided to stay in my equally precarious 7-year partnership.

Adam and I had tried saying goodbye to each other in vain several times before, but with so much distance between us now, this time seemed like it might actually take. He would have stayed if I'd asked him to, but how could I trust my feelings when we barely knew each other? Had I just conjured up the illusion of love as an excuse to end things with Peter? Was Adam just a cool, thirsty mirage in my noncommittal desert of tender but lukewarm adequacy?

At Against the Stream not long ago I'd asked one of my dharma teachers, Matthew Brensilver, how one might know which path to choose when each seemed equally uncertain. After a contemplative pause, he replied that in his own experience, the truest answers tend to arise as a simple and often quiet but definitive *YES* or *NO*. All I ever could hear bubbling up in my meditative silences was *I don't know I don't know I don't know*, like the scratchy crackle at the end of a record I couldn't decide whether to flip over or throw out the window.

Before Adam came along I'd lusted after an incredibly gifted and married classical musician named Robert. I *craved* him in a way I'd never craved another human being before. Over a series of casual meetups at restaurants and wine bars around town, I discovered we shared at least two things in common: a deep love of music, and the struggle of having a brilliant, devoted partner who you no longer connected with physically or romantically but couldn't bring yourself to say goodbye to. As author Elizabeth Gilbert had once described her first marriage: *'The only thing more unthinkable than leaving was staying; the only thing more impossible than staying was leaving.'* I would gaze at Robert on stage as he handled his instrument with intense precision, imagining those hands maneuvering their way beneath my blouse and pulling down my jeans.

"The investigation concluded that with multiple women, Mr. Levine violated the Third Precept of the Teacher's Code of Ethics, namely, 'to avoid creating harm through sexuality.' Events such as this have the power to shake one's confidence in the refuge of Buddha, Dharma and Sangha. We hope that the pain of this moment actually leads us back towards the heart and that we might all find true refuge..."

The first time Robert kissed me I'd just finished a glass of whiskey on the rocks and played one of Chopin's Preludes for him on the vintage baby grand in his foyer. My back was pressed against the wall near his large bay windows and his lips felt awkward, unable to sync with my rhythm. The second time Robert kissed me my back was pressed against the breasts of our mutual girlfriend under the sheets and his lips felt like the only thing I ever wanted on mine. I don't recall thinking about his wife or my boyfriend, only that we were too mortal to deny ourselves this blazing sense of aliveness that I'd forgotten I was capable of feeling. Some days it was all I could think about, the relentless beating of an aching melody I couldn't get out of my head.

I experienced a very different kind of yearning when Adam and I were introduced by a mutual friend at a gallery. It brewed slowly, beginning with our first meeting alone at a cafe where he confessed his struggles with bipolar disorder and I told him all about my own diagnosis after a manic episode in my twenties that was followed by months of debilitating depression. I cared greatly for him immediately and wanted to share the tools I used to stay grounded, the most foundational tool being a lifelong mindfulness meditation practice. I invited him to join me at Against the Stream, as I'd invited many friends and acquaintances before, to see if this practice might help him navigate his own waves of ups and downs.

By springtime Adam confessed he had strong feelings for me, and I realized mine were just as powerful for him. I'd always sensed that I was capable of loving this deeply – we had a connection that felt other-worldly, inspiring passionate poetry and songwriting, a recognition of paths having crossed many lifetimes before but perhaps never fully converging. We were aligned in so many ways, but Adam had a moral compass that my decades of dharma practice somehow failed to instill in me (or that I'd become so proficient at ignoring it may as well have been nonexistent). When that moral compass drove his decision that we couldn't be friends anymore, the grief left an ache so cavernous I felt certain only a relationship with God could fill it. I was wholly unprepared for the devastation that was still to come.

"With deep sadness, we announce that ATS will close the doors to its Melrose, Santa Monica and San Francisco centers on Sept 30, 2018... Though ATS is ending, the Dharma, as always, continues. The ripples and resonances of goodness and sincerity continue."

When our refuge and recovery sanctuary crumbled to the ground, my heart felt crushed by the weight of the wreckage. Noah Levine had guided and supported me in L.A. through the confusion of coming down from mania after my bipolar diagnosis, but I hadn't seen him in years. I knew the wisest among us could fall victim to our blind spots, so Noah's behavior didn't shake my faith in the dharma, but what about those who were newer to the community, who had sought shelter in a supposedly safe space to heal their own sexual trauma? Would they never again find comfort in the Buddha's teachings after realizing that those who shared them could still inflict so much harm?

Upon reaching Black Rock City, one of the first spaces I visited was Galaxia, the playa temple constructed of 20 timber trusses converging in a spiral towards the sky. I took slow steps towards the center mandala, desert dust caked in every orifice, and collapsed into myself as the tears wouldn't stop flowing. In 29 months, I would finally begin to grapple with the destructive impact of my own untempered sexual desires and misconduct: the devastation of betraying Adam's trust when he was finally ready to give his heart to me fully, and the painful confession to Robert's wife that we'd had an affair. In 9 weeks, my boyfriend and I would be clutching each other and sobbing as he asked if I really wanted to end our relationship, still ignorant (though not for long) to the ways I had been unfaithful. In 6 days, Matthew would be consoling our sangha during one of Against the Stream's final gatherings, my last visit to the Folsom Street Center that had become a second home to so many of us. As I reached the entrance I noticed the words "Me Too" sprayed in large black letters across the outside of the building. We listened intently to Matthew as we reckoned with this teaching of impermanence. "If 'Me Too' burned down our house," he said to us solemnly, "then maybe it needed to burn."

'From the moment I was six I felt sexy. And let me tell you it was hell, sheer hell, waiting to do something about it.' My eyes widened in recognition the first time I read this quote from silver screen siren Bette Davis. I was about 7 years old when I began grinding my hips against pool jets, and friends described me as "boy crazy" for as long as I can remember. I was enamored with unrequited new crushes easily and often throughout middle school and high school. It was rare that anyone showed interest in me, most notably a skinny kid with glasses and fluffy curls who approached me in the middle of the quad my freshman year and declared: *"I want to go out with you and I don't care that my friends say you're ugly."* It did nothing to boost my fragile self-esteem.

I got my first kiss in college, and after years of painful trial and error I eventually discovered that asking cute strangers *"Would I get in trouble if I tried to kiss you?"* was an obnoxiously easy and effective way to break the ice when you're a late bloomer trying to make up for lost time. I never dreamed I would get so much male attention when I was growing up and getting in trouble with my mom for leaving Ken and Barbie entwined in a naked embrace, or for using my Storybook computer program to position characters in Bacchanalian orgy scenes to my father's shock and horror.

In 2009, around the same time that I began an affair with another woman's boyfriend, I started an online project called *FKMYSELF.COM, A Celebration of Self Love*. It was meant to be a safe space for people to anonymously share their stories about sexual exploration and discovery, my attempt at taking a stand against societal stigmas and the patriarchal double standards that lead to women being slutshamed for daring to enjoy as many casual one-night stands as men do. I wanted to spark meaningful dialogue in a forum that didn't take itself too seriously. As fodder for my sex positive manifesto, a friend gave me her copy of Dossie Easton and Janet Hardy's *The Ethical Slut*, which challenged cultural norms about sex and relationships in its exploration of non-monogamy. I was inspired and emboldened by its message, but failed to finish the book or absorb the importance of the "Ethical" part of the practices.

Finally feeling desirable to men I desired gave me a hollow kind of validation that I had craved after painful years of awkward, lovelorn adolescence. It also fed my thirst and curiosity for a wide breadth of sensual connection, but it was easy to lose balance and act on impulse rather than out of integrity. I invented all kinds of reasons to justify why what I was doing in the moment was okay – societal boundaries constraining women's sexual freedom were meant to be broken; life was too short not to occasionally break the rules; giving myself what my partner couldn't understand I needed (because I didn't tell him) would ultimately save our relationship. None of these reasons would have held up under my own scrutiny or anyone else's.

It wasn't until I was forced to face the consequences of lying to myself and to men in my life who I supposedly cared for that I understood the importance of the Buddhist precepts of non-harming, which include refraining from taking what is not given, refraining from causing harm through sexuality, and refraining from lying or harmful speech. When I saw the deep suffering caused by my recklessness, the ways sexual misconduct destroys not only relationships but tears apart entire communities, I had to examine the selfishness and entitlement that drove the unconscious cruelty of my actions and identify the ways dishonesty showed up not just in my love life but occasionally my friendships and professional life too. *Wherever you go, there you are.*

I'd had my heart broken before, but nothing compared to the torment of seeing someone I love in such anger and agony as a result of my actions. All of my houses had burned to the ground. I knew that fully opening to the pain of remorse was a vital part of this lesson I needed to learn so that I would never repeat these mistakes again, but the shame and self-hatred that arose, focused on me instead of the impact I'd had on others, did not serve anyone. Noah had told me once that there is just as much ego in feeling small as there is in feeling great – both are just opposite sides of the same self-centered coin. He may have been wrong about many things, but I knew he was right about that. I struggled with insomnia for months and fell into a crisis of identity, not so different from the one I'd experienced in the months following my bipolar diagnosis when I wasn't sure how to distinguish the "real" parts of myself from my disorder. How could I have possibly shared the Buddha's teachings with so many but been blind to my inability to live by them?

I remembered attending a Vipassana meditation group with my parents the year of my manic episode when I was back home in Honolulu on medical leave from work. The group was led by a visiting monk from Southeast Asia at a local Buddhist temple. There was a period of guided sitting, followed by a talk and a short question and answer session. I raised my hand to ask him: *"How do I know who I am, when who I am always seems to be changing?"* The monk smiled and reminded me: *"The idea of having any solid self is the biggest illusion of all."* The only real constant in our experience is consciousness itself, the present observer of all the changing mental thoughts, feelings and sensations that flow through us day in and day out. This is what we can connect to and begin to see clearly in stillness. We can separate the mental chatter and judging mind from what is actually happening inside us and around us right here, right now. This is where we can find our inner peace, a harbor from the emotional storms. Fully present awareness, seeing and being with our experience just as it is, is the pathway to deliverance from our groundless imagined selves and our suffering.

One of my teachers, Vinny Ferraro, spoke to me once about the false refuges so many of us seek out – sex, drugs, food, money. It's easy to fall into a pattern of avoiding radical honesty and self-examination, choosing instead to numb or hide from the feelings and messages begging for our attention and healing. I had done this for far too long in many of my relationships, looking for a temporary fix or easy high instead of having the courage to initiate an authentic and difficult conversation about what both of us truly wanted and needed. In this way I had failed to love myself or anyone else. How can there be true love without truth and integrity?

The road to self-forgiveness was a difficult one, and I still experience moments of shame and regret, but I always strive to meet them with mindfulness and compassion. I sit in meditation, sometimes in front of a mirror, and bring non-judging awareness to of all my thoughts and sensations, to the witnessing of my perfectly imperfect parts. In tough moments I send myself Metta (loving kindness), silently whispering the phrases: *May I be at ease, May I be happy*, or turn to Ho'oponopono, a Hawaiian practice of reconciliation, repeating to myself and to those I've hurt: *I'm sorry, please forgive me, thank you, I love you.* I carve space almost daily for the simple joy of a one-woman silent disco party, putting on my headphones while my husband is still asleep, flipping my hair and shaking my limbs wildly in the morning sunshine on our wooden deck. I separate my inherent worthiness from the stories about my unskillful actions and take comfort in the Buddha's words from the Dhammapada: *"He who having been heedless is heedless no more, illuminates this world like the moon freed from clouds."* By seeing and owning my own shadow fully, accepting myself as I am and dedicating myself to non-harming, I'm better equipped to serve others and meet them in their own darkness with greater understanding.

Entering my forties as a happily married and monogamous woman, I'm learning to fully embrace my sensuality in healthier ways and let go of any constraints placed on that vital part of my being that arise from the fear of losing balance again and causing pain or instability in my partnership. Focusing my curiosity on *my own desire* instead of the need to *be desired* by others is a new adventure, and what I crave now more than anything is not a wide variety of carnal experiences but a deep, spiritual connection in my erotic life, one that is only possible through fully present, loving awareness. Where I once sought a misguided sexual freedom that disregarded the sanctity of my word and the feelings of others, I'm searching for a sensual, fully embodied, soul-nourishing liberation. When I'm grounded in my body instead of lost in my head, letting go of judgment and thoughts of the past or future, tuning into the warmth of my husband's skin and these precious breaths as if they might be my last, I'm able to be fully free.

About Kim Lange (Huynh)

Kim Lange (Huynh) is an award-winning filmmaker, photographer, and event curator from Honolulu, Hawai'i. She is passionate about cultivating meaningful, authentic connections in both large and intimate spaces, and fostering mental wealth in creative communities and beyond. Kim also serves on the Board of Mental Health Heroes and on the Advisory Board of Art With Impact, a nonprofit that promotes mental wellness by creating opportunities for young people to learn and connect through art and media. She has been practicing Vipassana (Insight) Meditation for over 25 years and began teacher training in 2023 through Jack Kornfield and Tara Brach's Mindfulness Meditation Teacher Certification Program with the Greater Good Science Center at UC Berkeley.

Follow her musings @kimalange

'We lose our sensual selves at the expense of ourselves because we must keep ourselves safe.'

- Carrie Myers

SUPPRESSING THE SENSUAL FOR SAFETY

by Carrie Myers

I recently watched the movie, *Confession*, (directed by Dayna Hanson, 2022) with my husband. The storyline was about a lady seeking justice for a gang rape. Ultimately, she gets her justice. However, this movie spoke loudly to me about sensuality. In cases of female sexual assault, victim blaming often becomes the excuse for an attack, but also creates a foundation for hiding our sensuality.

When a woman asks for help in seeking justice for a sexual assault, she is often questioned about what she was wearing. Was she showing too much skin? Was she drinking or experimenting with drugs at the time? Was she flirting and inviting sexual advances? Was she dancing provocatively? And so many more accusatory questions.

Only 18% of the adult women who are raped ever report the assault. One out of six American women have been a victim of attempted or successful rape in their lifetime (Rainn.org). But yet, the responsibility remains on women to prevent rape or other forms of sexual assault.

*Yet, we ask why women are disconnected
from their sensuality? Really?*

Are we seriously that oblivious?

My first question is how is it that the big, strong masculine has no control over himself once he is aroused? Why are women responsible for his **reaction** to their bodies? How is it that men have little to no responsibility for their reaction to a beautiful and sexy woman?

However, women "should" take care of themselves, have a great body and be eye candy for our men. We should do our nails and makeup to enhance our beauty. Women should be hair free and have smooth glowing skin. Women should also cater to the man's every need and whim...

BUT...

Don't be too sexy. Don't show off too much smooth and glowing skin. Wear the sexy dress, and heels, but don't move in a sexy manner such that will garner "unwanted" an "unwelcome" advances from men.

*Again, why can men not control themselves?
Why are women always in a battle of too much
and not enough, all at once?*

So, we hide our sensual side. We hide our desire. We hide our sexual trauma. We hide from our innate, authentic, beautiful, sensual, feminine selves.

Why? Because men cannot control their own sexual urges?

As we hide, we get more out of balance. We begin to edge our way into a more masculine way of being...

BECAUSE?

Because it is **our responsibility** to keep ourselves safe and safeguard ourselves from the "childish" way that men have been socialized to not be fully responsible for their masculine and sexual urges.

SO...

We lose our sensual selves at the expense of ourselves because we must keep ourselves safe. We cannot depend on the self-control from men who think that just because skin is displayed it is theirs for the taking, or the men who somehow feel like they had a right to react from their arousal as opposed to being in control of themselves.

In this confusing and mortifying world, where women are supposed to be sexy and in control, we are sent mixed messages in our role as women. We are supposed to be strong and in control, but we are supposed to be the "weaker" sex and submit to the men in the world. With this confusion, it is no wonder that we lose our sensuality and our flow and what is our innate wisdom and power as a feminine entity. We do want to be sexy and desirable, but we also want to be safe, respected and honored within our beauty and flow.

So, the question remains, how do we, as women, live from our sensual souls and still keep ourselves safe?

I do not have the answers to this ongoing battle. I do not know if women will ever be safe to fully express ourselves regardless of where we are, how we are dressed or how we dance. I do want to continue to keep this conversation and awareness spotlighted. I also strongly encourage us to keep each other safe and watch out for our sisters when we are out having fun. Stay safe, my sisters, while cheering each other on and protecting each other from the possible battles we may face.

'She is a force of reckoning'

- Carrie Myers

WOMAN ON FIRE
by Carrie Myers

She is not elusive
She is Bold
Never doubt her will
As her dreams unfold

Not just a spark
Nor a gentle candle glow
She is hot, bright, intense
As her fire continues to grow

Only few can handle
Her blazing aura and gaze
Only few can get close
To her stoked, yellow blaze

She isn't a woman
Who is an object of desire
She is a force of reckoning
This Woman On Fire

She Said Connection

by Carrie Myers

She said "connection"
He said "sex"
They were aiming at different destinations
No wonder they couldn't find each other

'I have found that seeking pleasure with purpose is the ticket...
Pleasure can be a powerful opening
to a loving connection with yourself - and others.'
- Laurie Riedman

THE PLEASURE PRACTICE
by Laurie Riedman

I've crossed the line. Have you?

For decades, I've been working on being able to experience and appreciate pleasure. No, not just the kind in the bedroom (or wherever you can snag that type of pleasure) – but the feeling of experiencing the joy of life's pleasures.

Inhabiting your true self fully in the moment.

Oh, and when you can do that "in the bedroom", you get extra points :)

> *'The moment is not found by seeking it,*
> *but by ceasing to escape from it.'* – James Pierce

Many of us have been conditioned to think that seeking pleasure is self-indulgent.

We have been taught that it's selfish.

It isn't.

Pleasure is inextricably married to our sense of aliveness and is hard-wired in us as humans.

Brain science shows us that we have pleasure centers in the midbrain. These are where our basic needs of food, sex, and physical exercise feed our emotions. Meeting these needs sends chemicals into our system, such as dopamine and serotonin, reinforcing that what we are doing feels good and urges us to do it again.

If this sounds familiar – unfortunately, this chain reaction is the root of many addictions. For example, for me, eating ice cream was something we did as a special treat as a child, so to this day, when I pass a soft serve stand – regardless of if I am hungry or not – I want it. I really, really want that ice cream.

By giving into that craving, I do feel the anticipatory sense of pleasure – pulling me toward it as I wait in line, deciding which flavor to get... and as I hold that twisted mound of cold, creamy deliciousness in my hand, I am feeding all my pleasure centers and reinforcing the pattern once again.

Unfortunately, I've conditioned my brain to "need" ice cream so that I can feel that chemical spike fueling that lovely level of satisfaction when I eat it.

The problem for me is that I forget that once I eat it, my tummy doesn't feel so good, and it doesn't fill me with pleasure.

Yet, my logical brain doesn't stand a chance when my reptilian brain sets that craving in motion. All it cares about is that I get the "high" my pleasure centers need, so I give in to the yearning. Willpower doesn't stand a chance as the magnetic pull of that soft serve wins, and I succumb and fulfil my desire for it lick by lick. This is an excellent example of confusing pleasure with comfort.

We have to define each of these for ourselves, but consider the following:

Comfort is soothing, distracting, calming, and healing.

Pleasure is enjoyable, rewarding, exciting, and fun.

I won't go into it here, but if you are interested in the spiritual teachings on this, you can check out *The Katha Upanishad*: ancient Hindu teachings that suggest that the wise will choose good over comfort. While there is so much more in these teachings, one lesson is that it is wise to try to go for depth rather than superficiality and ease.

This teaching is what I help my clients do – to do the "work" to get inside what truly is a pleasure for you by going deeper into self-awareness, learning to savor and surrender to pleasure.

'May we learn to be like a river that dances and sings the songs of the eternal, traveling and surrendering to the many bends until she finally meets her beloved ocean.'
– The Mundaka Upanishad

This has been my work for decades.

Pleasure was uncomfortable. I didn't know what it felt like. I couldn't be in the moment. Pleasure was the Holy Grail for me for most of my adult years.

As a survivor of childhood sexual abuse, I've had to learn what I want, what makes me feel good – inside and out.

And to allow myself to go there.

I've had to learn how to meet those needs. To practice asking for what I need and want (even if they are different). This lesson has probably been the hardest to learn of all!

I have had to train my brain that those signs that I am experiencing pleasure in my body do not need to sound an alarm anymore. It has taken decades to learn how to short-circuit the automatic "danger, danger" signals my brain would send, instantly transporting me in nanoseconds into a confused and frightened child of about five or six.

Years ago, as my husband and I were working on our intimacy issues, carefully navigating the automatic land mines of my brain's survival instinct, I would experience these short-circuit moments with no warning.

One particular evening, I was slightly annoyed and blinded by the light shining from the bathroom as I waited for Rich, my husband of 33 years, to finish at the sink and come to bed. Then it happened. Glancing out of the corner of my eye, I noticed his backlit, semi-nude male body silhouetted in the doorway. My brain didn't skip a beat as my retina registered the image, and I immediately gasped and held my breath as adrenaline and fear gripped my body.

In milliseconds, I'm no longer a wife waiting for the man she loves to crawl into bed but a child in my twin bed in my bedroom on the second floor of my childhood home. I'm gripping the sheets with my fingers, simultaneously squeezing my eyes shut, hoping to trick "him" into thinking I'm asleep.

These triggered moments happened frequently as I worked with professionals – and my patient and loving husband – to learn how to stay in the present moment. Eventually, those time-traveling triggers began to happen less and less. Slowly, my husband and I mapped out how my body could experience pleasure as if we were explorers navigating unknown territory. It was scary and fun.

Decades later, I can safely say this 60-plus-year-old woman is one hot, sexy mama who loves – and even seeks – pleasure in all areas of my life.

I have found that seeking pleasure with purpose is the ticket.

It's a subtle difference. We can seek and find sensual pleasure, loving intimacy, action with purpose and passion, creativity, and deep spirituality in eating a decadent piece of chocolate cake and the loving embrace of a loved one. I find this level of pleasure in watching a glorious sunset or a child jumping in a mud puddle after a storm.

Pleasure can be a powerful opening to a loving connection with yourself – and others. But I have found that I first had to find pleasure within myself to find pleasure with others.

Writing has become a source of immense pleasure for me. I get lost in the words and in the moment of writing, only to stop and realize I've been at my computer for hours. Have you ever gotten lost in joyful moments – just moments – yet felt like time stopped and it felt longer? Or sat watching a bird build a nest or waves on the water and suddenly noticed the sun was going down? Time stops when we are in such a profound experience.

When my clients have trouble accessing pleasure, we begin by taking time to discover what brings them joy – and we seek out those moments and prioritize those activities. If you don't know what this might be – when do you feel inspired? What makes you smile on the inside and out? When was the last time you felt joy – or witnessed pure joy?

These can offer hints about where to find this type of personal pleasure.

Sensual pleasure can include the taste of fantastic food, the smell of a summer beach rose, or getting lost in a piece of art. These delights stimulate the same pleasure centers as the desire we feel anticipating the touch of our loved ones.

I've learned to train myself to stay physically present with my body so I can feel that delight. I've had to untrain protective habits I learned as a self-defensive mechanism when I was younger being abused. I left my body in those moments to survive. I've worked so hard to be present to feel deep pleasure in those moments. I am grateful I can do this more often than not.

I am happy I've learned how to bring my pleasure centers back online after being hidden from me for years.

I can re-ignite my pleasure centers and stay in my body with attention and patience. I practiced this by staying aware of simple pleasures – indulging in an expensive piece of dark chocolate or getting a massage and genuinely feeling the bliss as my muscles relaxed.

Let's take the sensual pleasure of eating to explore this. Tying this lesson to eating has been an excellent way to play with and discover sensual pleasure because eating can be a desirable experience. And that isn't bad. Don't get lost in shame or guilt if you are present with it.

Whether you are eating freshly picked dew-covered berries or being aroused by your loved one's touch, if we focus on the sensations we are feeling, we can find our way to get lost in pleasure. Here is how I've done it.

1. Take a breath and focus on the sensation of the moment – the feeling of the touch or perhaps the taste of what you are eating.

2. Focus on what you are feeling rather than what has triggered that feeling. Stay with the feeling.

3. Let the sensation expand. Let it grow. (I have found it helps to think of where I feel that sensation in my body and like I'm using my GPS to click in and expand closer – I click in and focus inward more.)

4. Stay with it, and soon you will feel as if a tiny bubble has burst – just a slight letting go of pressure – and you will be opening the door of pleasure – even just a little bit.

5. The more you stay with it – the more the door will open to a new world of joy, beauty, love, grace, and _____ (you fill in the adjective that works for you!).

> *"What day is it?"*
> *"It's today," squeaked Piglet.*
> *"My favorite day," said Pooh.'* – A.A. Milne

I would love to hear how you feel pleasure in your life. What brings you joyful rapture in your life? What keeps you in the moment the longest?

Here's to the pursuit of pleasure! We crave it naturally but have to learn how to go for it. I guarantee I'll still stop for that soft serve and perhaps feel a momentary feeling of pleasure despite the future tummy ache. It's a work in progress, my friends.

Pleasure is a practice.

About Laurie Riedman

Laurie Riedman is a personal and relationship coach, writer, and storyteller. After thirty-five years running her own PR and marketing firm, she transitioned her consulting to coaching, founding b.u. coaching to support those – like her – who seek to embrace their truths and be their best selves in all aspects of their personal and professional lives.

Writing and publishing essays on her blog More Than Words and publishing her memoir Diamonds in the Dirt: Stories From a Junkyard Girl are part of her healing journey. She has also published essays in Bluff & Vine. Her writing is included in two anthologies – one she co-edited with Susan Walter titled Badass Sisterhood and the forthcoming Sensual Soul Shine.

Laurie lives, writes, and coaches from her home along Canandaigua Lake in the Finger Lakes of New York. Married to her life partner Rich for over 38 years, they have founded three successful companies and raised three amazing daughters: Elizabeth, Beck, and Hannah.

You can find out more about Laurie and her work on her website: www.laurieriedman.com

'When do we learn to mistrust our sensuality?'

- Nicola Humber

HOMECOMING
by Nicola Humber

I remember how it felt.

Walking into that theatre. Music ringing out. Women talking excitedly, finding a seat where they could land.

Others (like me) edging their way in, looking for safety, wanting to remain invisible for as long as possible.

I felt sick.

It was the first weekend of Mama Gena's Mastery program in New York City. I'd loved her book, *Pussy: A Reclamation* and after reading it, I'd tentatively checked out how to work with her in some way. So when a friend suggested attending her flagship Mastery program, I thought it was meant to be.

Yes. I'm in.

And then, a week or so beforehand, my friend discovered she wouldn't be able to travel after all. I was on my own.

'No problem' I told myself. I was used to travelling alone. It was only a short hop from where I was based in upstate New York. I'd been to a ton of personal development events in the past. How different could this be?

The answer: VERY different.

And as I walked in on that Saturday morning, I could feel it.

Hundreds of women gathered together.

All with the intention to connect more deeply with their pleasure.

The energy was thick, potent. It felt like I was pushing against something palpable as I tried to find a way to my seat.

Finding a spot, I sat next to a woman who immediately sniffed and said, *'Is that Pomegranate Noir?'*

My signature perfume. I loved it. How great to establish an immediate connection.

'Eurgh, I hate it. There's something about it that gives me a headache'.

Oh.

In this room of sisters, I'd managed to get it wrong somehow right off the bat.

'It's okay', she said, *'I'm sure it will be fine'*.

But I felt like the outsider deep down I knew I was.

I didn't belong here. That was clear.

Somehow I kept myself in my seat and forced myself to stay. You know when every cell in your being is telling you to run? That's how I felt. Somehow it felt unsafe to be in this place where other women were gathered. A part of me knew I was there for a reason though. I'd felt the call. I trusted that.

And later that morning, I found myself naked.

Yes, naked.

Mama Gena knows how to start her events with a bang and within the first hour or so of us arriving, she invited (or should I say challenged!) us to strip off. The intention was to connect with our bodies, to let ourselves be seen, to celebrate our glorious selves and have a Pussy Parade across the stage.

I don't know if it was my need to fit in, a reluctance to be one of the few women who didn't play along, or a true desire to let the fuck go, but I tore off my clothes (wishing I'd chosen better underwear) and danced around the room.

And although a part of me definitely felt uncomfortable, surprisingly another part, deep down, felt like she'd come home.

The feeling of communion in the room was stunning.

THIS is how it's meant to be.

Not necessarily that we have to spend every minute dancing naked together (although, maybe that wouldn't be a bad thing?) But the sense of connection, celebration, allowing our bodies to be seen, allowing our beings to be seen, and revelling in that, revelling in ourselves.

Yes.

But why did this feel like such a big step for me?

Why had I nearly run from this room before the event even started?

Why do we need 'training' to connect with our pleasure?

When do we learn to mistrust our sensuality?

For this, I need to take you back further. Back to when I was a teeny tiny girl, living in a council house in 70s England. I remember vividly the first time I realised that my body could be pleasure-full. Lying on my front I would rub the magic place between my legs and it felt AMAZING.

I thought I'd discovered the best secret ever. And of course I decided to take my fill of pleasure whenever I could.

My favourite spot was to position myself half under the sofa in the living room. Little Nicola would lie on the floor and rub her magic spot with abandon.

Life was good.

But then, my parents, who kinda ignored this for a little while, obviously realised there was no way I was growing out of this phase and told me, in no uncertain terms, that it wasn't acceptable.

I'm not sure exactly what they said. I'm sure they felt super-awkward, because no-one really talked about anything like 'that' back then. But I received the message loud and clear.

What I'd been doing was shameful.

It was NOT good to be enjoying myself in this way.

My pleasure was wrong.

And my body couldn't be trusted, especially my magic spot.

This was the beginning of a long journey where I learned that feeling good, feeling myself, BEING myself, was NOT what society was looking for.

I learned to keep my desires under wraps, a secret, even to myself.

I learned that being a good girl, putting others' needs before my own, getting good grades and toeing the line got me approval.

So for years that's what I did. Years and years.

Sensuality wasn't a consideration for me. I did well at school, went on to university, got a good job and followed the path I thought was expected of me.

But my sensual self would burst out every now and again in disruptive and sometimes risky ways. Relationships with the wrong men. Putting myself in dangerous situations.

Living with a guy who ended up in prison.

An affair with a married colleague.

I was a good girl with a wild side, but the wild side wasn't truly mine. It was a warped expression of all the desires I'd kept pushed down. I couldn't see that though. And I made myself wrong, over and over again, because I couldn't seem to stop making bad decisions.

What the frick was wrong with me?

It was only after changing my path, leaving my 'proper' job to retrain as a hypnotherapist, meeting my now husband and TRULY beginning to know myself, that I was able to reconnect with my sensuality in a healthy way.

When I entered the online space back in 2013, I suddenly started to find all of these women who were talking about the Divine Feminine. I realised that I'd been operating from my masculine for all this time, pushing through and ignoring my body. I'd subconsciously been seeing my

Feminine as weak and not to be trusted. After all, this aspect of me had done nothing but get me into trouble.

It was a long path back to rebuilding trust. Reading books, taking classes, even performing in a Burlesque show and gradually, gradually getting to know this part of me I'd forgotten and suppressed.

This culminated with my adventures at Mama Gena's Mastery. From that first Saturday, stripping off with strangers, letting myself be seen and seeing others, it was maybe the most transformational experience of my life.

Allowing my Feminine to lead the way.

Recognising that sensuality had (many) more than one side. One of the most potent experiences I had was allowing grief to move through my body whilst being witnessed by a small group of women. It felt deeply sensual and sacred.

Connecting with and allowing myself to be seen by the different women I met during my time at Mastery was life-changing. I'd never really allowed myself to fall fully into sisterhood, but the sense of us all uplifting each other in that space was potent.

What I realised is that sensuality isn't just a personal experience, or one we have with an intimate partner, it can be felt and celebrated in community too. Of course, as women we've been conditioned to see other women as a threat, as someone to compete with. The media leads the way when it comes to shaming, criticising and ridiculing any woman who dares to love on herself and be in her sensuality.

Being in sisterhood like this, perhaps for the first time, was so very liberating. On the last weekend when we were invited to dress as courtesans, expressing our sensuality in whatever way felt most powerful for us, the air of celebration was joyous.

Again it felt like coming home.

I'm so grateful for that experience of getting to attend Mama Gena's Mastery program.

I'm grateful for the way it shifted my relationship with myself and my sensuality.

And I'm grateful for how that relationship has continued to evolve over the past 5 years as I've moved from my forties into my fifties.

I guess Mama Gena has been an influence with this too? As a woman in her sixties, she's very much still rocking her sensual self. There's been no slipping away into invisibility as middle-aged and older women are generally trained to do.

As I've started to fully navigate the ageing process, rather than despairing of or resigning to the changes in my body, I've allowed myself (most of the time!) to celebrate them.

Yes, my belly is rounder.

Yes, my hair is silver rather than the dark brown it was in my twenties and thirties.

Yes, my breasts have swollen..

But I feel more comfortable in my skin than I ever have.

I don't feel the pressure to meet the expectations I did when I was a younger woman, carefully dyeing and straightening my hair, shaving my legs and armpits meticulously, keeping myself 'trim'.

Nope. I still very much care and tend to my incredible body, but she doesn't have to look a particular way.

I run my hands over my new-found curves, lumps and bumps.

I glory in my silver locks.

I honour the elder woman I'm becoming.

At home in my bones.

About Nicola Humber

Nicola Humber is the author of three transformational books, *Heal Your Inner Good Girl*, *UNBOUND* and *Unbound Writing* and creator of the *#unbound365 journal*. She's also the founder of The Unbound Press, a soul-led publishing imprint for unbound women.

After playing the archetypal good girl up until her mid-thirties, Nicola left her 'proper' job in finance to retrain as a coach and hypnotherapist and this leap of faith led her to what she does now: activating recovering good girls to embrace their so-called imperfections and shake off the tyranny of 'shoulds', so they can be their fullest, freest, most magnificent selves.

Nicola helps women to write the book their Unbound Self is calling them to write, whilst growing a community of soul-family readers and clients.

She's also the host of The Unbound Writer's Club podcast.

Find out more at: nicolahumber.com

'A ripple of Truth expressed and translated.
Sensual creativity seeded and mated.
Within us all is both the masculine and feminine.
Here come Sensual Souls birthing sensual creations.'
- Patricia Alessandra Levy

YOUR AUTHENTIC EXPRESSION
by Patricia Alessandra Levy

Bloom in Secret

Bursting open
Arms wide open
Chest strong
Core in stride

Leading and trusting,
your center is your guide.

Abundance, presence, creativity, and full expression.

They are all one in the same
Sensuality is simply
speaking of another part of the game.

Living, breathing,
Falling, believing.

Where this journey leads you are the moments
in-between.

Not the highlights,
but the lived in process.
The journey, this connecting, is the softening we need.

Bloom in secret, intimately true.
Sensual soul, it is a wave of being and receiving
the world as it is
exactly as you.

Sensual Creations

A ripple of Truth expressed and translated,
Sensual creativity seeded and mated.

Within us all is
both the masculine and feminine.

Here come Sensual Souls birthing sensual creations.

As I sat there, I wanted to understand so badly how I could.

How I could make it happen

How I could will it to become

And how I could easefully, openly, and gracefully allow the free flow to birth as one.

Creativity is a wondrous thing. It is a mystery and knowing in how it is to be done. I have spent so many years trying to figure it out. *How am I going to create what I came here to do? What is the thing I am here for?*

It was the strongest and most painful knowing to have this sense of purpose without any answers in regard to how or why. For many, this felt-sense may be recognized more for its trauma because it often leads us into doubt, frustration, and eventually hopelessness. It has a way of pointing out where and how we do not fit in. It definitely did for me, and I am sure it has for then some.

For it is in our rational-thinking world that we do not vocalize the transformation of a felt-sense path and because of this, many have not yet birthed into who they are meant to become.

The Dragonfly Emergence

While my journey has been like a dragonfly, with all its dips and turns, moltings and sudden emergence, I have found my sensuality to be the thing that gracefully opened me up to evolve through some very prompt and sudden ascension phases in my life. The kind which require immense awareness and bravery to align my creative process and bring my entire life into one.

As nature speaks, the dragonfly is a unique creature compared to other winged insects, such as butterflies, as they do not have a cocooning stage between being a larva (nymph) and an adult (dragonfly). Living in the water most of their nymph life, nymphs experience multiple moltings (also noted as generations) of their body before their final molt to become a dragonfly.*

How many lifetimes do we often experience as we grow with our bodies? The resonance that this speaks brings me to think of all the identities and generations of myself I have experienced as a maiden. The number seems countless and dizzying. The dips and turns of this part of my life were incredibly unwinding. They brought me to remember the most sacred parts of me.

When the dragonfly is ready to complete its final molt, it will wait for the environment to relay the perfect conditions. With no surprise, spring's longer days and warmer temperatures are the nymph's choice. This is nature's alignment. Spring is almost always the perfect environment for a body to express itself into full emergence.

As I write this, I am moving through a pivotal passage of winter, both within and without. A cold front has moved through the valley of our desert home and my daughter, mother and I have just recently celebrated our solar returns: 3 years, 60 years, and 30 years young respectively. Three is the number of harmony, support and balance between the mind, body and spirit. While six is the number of introspection. With these numbers, we reveal the greatest invitation of winter: to find harmony in your journey of introspection.

For me, this is always my experience in winter. Pivotal yet harmonious wayfinding, especially this year. Across many dimensions (mother, wife, daughter and creatress), there is an abundance that I am moving through with a horizon that reveals new eras of adventure opening up for me. However, as the dragonfly waits to emerge at the cusp of Spring, I too have found a cultivation of power in waiting through winter.

When the final molt is ready to occur, the nymph will find herself in shallow water and attune her body to breathe in air. Then slowly, she will begin to pull herself out of her skin with only one 30-minute pause in between her upper and lower half. When her body is fully out in the open, her core and wings will expand leaving behind a cast. Her first flight as a dragonfly is short in length and incredibly vulnerable, and yet even so, her emergence is complete.

The maturation of your spirit always brings a natural rhythm of newness and youthful adventure. The polarity of growing wiser is the accumulation of more youth behind your eyes. When we are honest and in connection with the roots of ourselves, the grounded and uplifted creations of Self will be what emerges.

In my own journey of nymph to dragonfly, remembering this way of sensual creation was the culmination of my final molt.

Know the Flow

Here we define sensuality as a means of opening up your senses (sight, smell, hearing, touch, and inner sense) and sensual creation as receiving and being guided by what you feel and what *speaks* up. With that in mind, to better understand how sensuality plays a role in your ability to create with heart and intention, it is helpful to first learn how the energy exists and flows through your body.

In Eastern theory, there is a word for your True Essence and the movement it takes both within and without your body. This word is called 'Chi' and it represents life force energy.** Life force energy ultimately illuminates your dynamic relationships to life. How you relate to yourself, to others, the sensations, thoughts, emotions, physicality of your body and everything that exists in your life is expressed as the movement and quality of your Chi. Like the wind that speaks to the birds as they migrate from place to place, Chi is the Universal presence of everything that becomes and just is.

Life is ever-changing and there is never a ceasing moment when things, no matter how stable they may seem, are not shifting form. Your Chi represents both your form and formless nature. So, while there is a whole world that exists in a particularly designed way (e.g. your body, your unique way of thinking, your ancestry, habitual patterns, etc.) there is also a True Essence of You that exists in formlessness (universal creation, nonduality, and pure consciousness). This is one of the reasons why meditation, self-reflection, and energetic mind-body awareness is so supportive for your wellbeing. As you become more aware of the movement and expression of your Chi, you will broaden your understanding and relationships to Self.

Now, Let's Talk Sensual Creation

Your sensuality is your Chi expressed in form. It reveals the flow of your True Essence and relays your authentic expression. Your body is a beautiful vessel receiving life as it most Divinely moves through and with you. So, again to define sensuality, it is to open your senses and allow the movement of life force energy to enter you. And then, to sensually create, is to co-create with this greater relationship to both formlessness and form.

To further put this into words, imagine yourself sitting at a kitchen table facing a tall window. Sensual openness is allowing the music from the other room to penetrate you. It is to see the white and wispy ice on the driveway across the way. And, it is to feel the keys of your computer heavy beneath your hand. The words start to flow as everything around you moves through you one in the same. Maybe, your ears will pick up a special tone or word sung. Maybe your eyes will be drawn to a particular color in the room. These sparks may influence your creation. Whatever it may be, your creativity will reflect this universal movement and cohesion of everything around you. The difference that this creation will make will be powerful and intentional.

All embodying, allowing, and timeless.

Sensual creations are impactful because when you are open to receiving, you are co-creating with the life force energy present both in and beyond the room. Your sensuality draws in on how you relate to the world around you, an expression of your True Essence. To recognize this, let us imagine all of the most moving works of art that were created in times of strife, hardship, and struggle. Imagine what the artists of these pieces were receiving through their senses and how the translation of their True Essence imprinted an impact.

With this said, the Universe, if not entirely, will synchronistically and divinely support you to trust in your sensuality and birth creations. More sensual art needs to be made in this world. More sensually-led lives need to be embodied. And more, sensually empowered people need to be in their presence.

Healing & Gaining Trust

I will now shed light on the stickiness that comes when we are learning to trust in our senses. With any sort of movement, there will be a season of stagnation and blocks. That is the natural order in our journey of bringing our world into balance. The opportunity is what exists in challenge and while the abundant nature of Chi is to flow, flow, and flow. We all experience our own trials and tribulations when it comes to our sensual flow.

As I write that, I start to experience a wave of self-criticism and hear thoughts on what may or may not have been the cause of my own personal blocks I had experienced in the past. I want to blame others and myself for the disconnect I had felt so long in my own body. It is easy to assume energy blockage can mean something is bad or wrong.

"If my energy is blocked then I must be doing something wrong."

However, in these moments, it is beautiful to remember the constrictions and contractions that are there to heighten our awareness. *"Yes! Please speak louder because I did not know it was you who was speaking"* were words I have told my own life and body.

Stagnation and blockages are necessary fuel that we use to molt all the generations of ourselves before we reach our finale emergence. They identify portals of activation and connection that will be foundational in our creations years to come.

When I was in my own moltings and shedding generations of myself, I was taking baby steps in reclaiming myself as a sensual creatress. I had moved through limitations in owning my own desires, voice and body, healed sisterhood wounds and learned womb wisdom, found independence in pleasure, and listened to my senses with a sacred yet playful reverence. Every single one of these opportunities came from a stagnation and block, and while it was a rollercoaster to experience them one after another, each one had its purpose and ultimately set me up.

In my eyes, my finale molt came after I cultivated a deeper and fuller acceptance for presence in myself and my life. A finale that truly lives up to its name. For, it was not until I embodied the connection of sensual presence did my creativity begin to play a higher game.

With gratitude, this teaching was bestowed upon me via my 2-year-old daughter, Ayla.

Sensuality and Parenting

When I reawakened my sensual appetite, I had fully immersed myself as a stay-at-home parent and embarked through the trolls of reparenting my unworthiness blues. This idea of reparenting illuminates the journey one goes through when they are taking care of a child or elder.

When Ayla was 2, her energy brought up a lot around duality for me.

This is true about the potency of the number two, which brings up the wisdom on duality. Duality tells us that we can have either this or that and it is either black or white. If we are in one opposite extreme, then the latter must be at fault.

Humanity has a funny way of rooting ourselves in these categories of opposites. So that when we do not see eye to eye, obtaining harmony is quite difficult. However, as a *terrible 2-year-old* exhibits, we really do not like the idea of separation and there is an innate rebuttal when life makes us think that it must be this or that way.

With that said, unity is a strong message that comes with the energy of two. Here, I felt a wave of reconsideration. All the ways I held myself and my life in criticism, judgment, and anger because it was this and not that bubbled to surface. Ayla's energy mirrored to me the parts of myself that I judged so uncompassionately. Therefore, the terrible-ness in 2 is not from the child running rampage herself, and instead it is from the energy of Truth that her pureness of age brings up for the caregiver or parent.

It was at this time of my life, when it all felt incredibly pivoting, chaotic and highly dynamic, that my sensuality sprung itself forward to help me out. While my inner world was colliding with all sorts of emotional and psychological distress, I had absolutely no clue what to do in regard to my direction: *How do I parent? Where in the world is our life going from here? And stomping my feet, what is the point?!*

My sensuality provided me with both the answers and the means of establishing connection. Not only did I start to understand what it truly meant to be present, but I found myself gauging my senses as a guide as to whether or not I was open and receiving my life. This helped me tremendously in making everyday decisions to better take care of myself and my family. Amidst the potent lessons on duality, my senses led me to find acceptance. I chose to see in wholeness instead of separation and I found this hidden power in creating my life from this felt-sense.

Creating From a Felt Sense: Reimagine Channeling

Channeling is full presence in the body. It is a connection between the heart, mind and Spirit.

It is taking life by submerging yourself one step at a time, feeling the air as it breezes across your face and feet, to look someone in the eye and catch where they are at by the pace of their breath, understanding body language, empathizing and delivering yourself with confidence, clarity and heart-led connection.

When it comes to what channeling is and what it looks like, there is so much to be understood. And quite frankly, the spectrum of it as an action or way of being ranges quite a lot. Additionally, it may be more shocking and difficult to grasp channeling when you are witnessing another person doing it. For instance, I remember my first experience seeing a sister of mine *channel* at a retreat. Moments prior to her starting, I felt nothing out of the ordinary, and then only the slightest of sensations shifted and the hairs raised on my arm. I listened to her with my heart. However, as soon as she *completed her oracular message*, it was like clockwork. My mind instantly boggled, I was utterly confused and my thoughts immediately were in dispute.

I soon learned afterwards that I simply needed a reason to trust. Trust in the unimaginable and lean into what I was sensing. Everything my body replayed from that moment felt pure, intentional and real. Everything my thoughts wanted to rage about was rooted in fear. Evidently, this is where I had to make a choice, illuminating the ultimate power of your sensuality: empowerment.

Empowerment has been my greatest choice in life. When I began to understand my choices in regard to opening up to my senses, I chose the path of least resistance and unconditional love to result in more *openness*. I wanted to trust in the unimaginable and lean into the things that tasted, smelt, felt or I just knew to be pure and intentional. This became my road map to creating: a blend of dreamy, raw, and real.

Channeling is a Miraculous Unfolding of Life

It is an integrated and embodied expression of Love. When we speak with the integrity of what truly lives within our hearts, we start to obtain *information* that encourages a radiance of this *flow*. Creation will unfold with joy and ease as opposed to the aggressive, overworked, over-stimulated, and disempowering ways sensual exploitation has ridiculed us to believe.

Embodied pleasure is completely shadowed out in many parts of the world. What is missing is an interweaving peace that will naturally envelope from within and bring you forward. A serendipitous bloom, a death and a sunrise all happening simultaneously at once.

Think of artists making music or software engineers coding. Animals, children, gate keepers. *We are all meant to be channels and bridges for this universal flow creating networks of consciousness into our lives and existence through our being of art.*

The Sensual Leaders

Comically, the ebbs and flows of life are always in all ways leading us to our most impactful creations. The play is in wondering: *are we really where we need to be?* In truth, we never really know what it is that our soul or another needs. So, connect with the energetic movements of life force energy, formally known as Chi, to become more self-conscious of your relationships. Because in order for one to make a conscious impact, they must be conscious of how life moves and engages with them.

In total simplicity, life is meant to be received and you are meant to be the receiver. What and how you receive is governed by your senses. And, your sensuality is your channeling.

As an ambitious leader, sensuality was a homecoming for me. I laugh now, because five years on my intuitive path, I thought I was doing the things, but there were so many lessons and reasons to trust before this new way of Sensual Creation became me. Acceptance, becoming a mother, abundance, presence, and being in the lived in process was where my sensorial practice truly became.

Ah, okay. This.
This is what is truly here.
This is how I create.
This is me.

The simple, the necessary, and the in-between. A timeless beacon for conscious creativity and empowered living lies in the choice of receiving and openness. This is the Divine Feminine through and through.

So, as you witness a collaboration of stories of the woman's journey of attuning to her senses, know that your story is both unique and that you are not alone. This message is for the woman who has always known deep down that there is something here for her to create in this lifetime as an expression of herself. Then, when the wombs of our world have forged their truth and spoken, no longer needing to restore the generations of sensuality shamed and outcasted, this message will call to the sensual creativity within us all.

The greater invitation lies in reclaiming the Divine Feminine in conscious creation. Sensuality, listening, blooming in secret, healing, transforming, and tuning in.

Sensual Soul, you are here to deepen and open.

What is alive and finally ready to come out from inside of you?

The world is ready.

May you feel the support of all that have journeyed before you.

Resources

*https://british-dragonflies.org.uk/odonata/life-cycle-and-biology/

**https://www.ekhartyoga.com/articles/practice/what-is-chi

About Patricia Alessandra Levy

Patricia Alessandra Levy is an author, healer, creatress and mother. Writing is her choice of channeling after she began opening up her senses and creating from this space of conscious connection. You may receive and support her work via her online newsletter, Oracle Delivery, via Oracledelivery.substack.com

'Magnetising all to her, multiplying... electrifying, orgasmic bliss, creative and inspired. Wisdom whispers softly now... Remember woman... Pleasure IS your Power!!!'

- Siobhan Gannon

UNSHACKLED: A RETURN TO EROTIC INNOCENCE

by Siobhan Gannon

Breaking the chains of generational silence; transforming trauma into spiritual liberation, body autonomy and erotic empowerment

Sensual Soul Shine is a beautiful, multifaceted phenomenon that celebrates life's essence and the intricate interconnectedness of mind, body and spirit.

Erotic Poetry... to ignite your senses, illuminate your soul and set your desires on Fire!!!

This poem captures the essence of making love before dawn, where shadows blend with light, symbolising a return to the unity of erotic innocence. It serves as a metaphor for the emergence of a New Earth and the harmonious integration of divine masculine and feminine energies within ourselves and in the world.

Twilight – A New Earth is Dawning

Moonlight, stillness
Starlight… windows glistening
Bedcovers shuffle
Soft moan…
Shh… He's stirring
His Lionheart rumbles
Sleepy yawns, erotic tingles

Light caresses
Skin to skin
Parted lips, fingertips
Sexy hips, tenderly touched
Soft kisses, erotic images…

Whispers softly in her ear
Commanding… desiring
Awaken for him
Nape of her neck
She feels that arousal
Hairs stand to attention
Bodies listening…
That's woman's empowerment

Hearts beat faster,
Slow breaths quicken
Inhale… exhale
Soul connections deepen

Rising passion from within
Her cauldron stirs
Womb fire burns
Embers gathered
Wild souls ecstatic
Liberated, intoxicated
Time to roam free again

She speaks
Slow and contemptuous
Awoken from her slumber now
Unbridled, lustful
Sweet soul surrender

Arousing eros
Hungry for power
Ripples in waves
Blood courses through her veins

Fiery heart opens
Illuminated and raw
Her desire, her fire
Enticing... inviting
Soully lit and potent
She burns like a woman
In her authentic aliveness!!

Can you feel her fullness now
Her soul ignited
Erotic... innocent
Divine and entitled

Desires on fire
Willing her to remember
Her sacred sensuality
Her potent feminine superpowers

Her yoni awakens
Moist and inviting
She's ready to receive
Orgasmic… enlightened
Her juices trickling from within
Her heart,
Her soul
Her womb
Her queen

Magnetising all to her
Multiplying, electrifying
Orgasmic bliss
Creative and inspired
Wisdom whispers softly now
Remember… woman…
Pleasure is your power

Sensual soul alive and ecstatic
Sexual endeavour
Potent and empowered
Magnifying, alluring
Pulsating, exciting

Bare breasts, hairy chest

Wild souls free again
Ah...
her breath, her fire
Exasperation... wholly complete
Lionheart roars
Relieved and released

Bodies relaxed now
Soft and surrendered
Senses tuned up
Immersed and uncensored

Erotic juices
Flowing as one
Bodies ravished
Hungers eradicated

Slow down, soft gaze
Satiated, intoxicated
Returned to their slumber
Blissful and complete
Contented, embodied
Souls are at peace

Whispers of *'I love you'*
Time has come for sleep
A new day is dawning
Morning's... just around the corner

In this chapter, I've chosen to share a deeply personal story that marked a significant turning point in my life. At the tender age of 18, this awakening had a profound impact on my self-perception as a spiritual, sensual and sexual young woman. And has been instrumental in shaping the empowered woman that I am today.

It was the beginning of a long and ever-evolving journey to recovery, moving through suppressed and repressed shame and guilt to reclaiming body autonomy, my sacred sensuality, and sexuality... my true erotic innocence, my essence and heart's desires.

Through my words, I invite you to find healing, solace, inspiration and encouragement as you step further into your own change journey towards autonomy, authenticity and self-empowerment.

Spiritual & Sexual Awakening

It was 2010 when I began exploring energy medicine as a natural approach to heal psoriatic arthritis, fibromyalgia and depression. For years I've equated this with my conscious spiritual and sexual awakening. However, upon reflection, in truth, it all began back in 1990 when I was just 18 years old. It was during my first year of college when an unplanned pregnancy and subsequent termination were going to change me and the trajectory of my life forever. A series of pivotal moments in time, that initiated my journey of awakening, True empowerment was to follow many, many years later…

My Story

As I write this piece, I'm transported back in time to 1990, recalling the moment I saw my first love…

The music was loud, the night still young. I felt the excitement inside building as the crowd flowed in. I remember something palpable in the air that night. I couldn't touch it… just a sense of surrender within.

A deep knowing perhaps, that a new chapter of my life was just about to begin…

We met on the stairs…

It was one of those love at first sight moments, where, you know… time stands still, and we soon ended up head over heels for each other, him for me and me for him… First love I guess you'd call it.

I'd just turned 18 that summer and had started my first year in college in the September. Savouring that first taste of freedom, living away from home and family.

Our romance was blossoming and feelings were alive and intense at times. College became less of a priority, partly because I wasn't enjoying my course and partly because he became my world...

I wasn't much of a multitasker... I loved to party, so it was often one or the other. I was the girl who never wanted the music to stop or the night to end.

So, I guess, all was well really in my romance bubble world and I didn't really contemplate life beyond that. I was very much living in the moment, day to day.

But that was all to change when one day out of the blue, a friend asked me to accompany her to a clinic for a pregnancy test. Despite not feeling well myself, I went to support and reassure her. Whilst there, I decided to take a test myself, more out of curiosity than concern, you know, just for the craic, as I had been using contraception.

What happened next sent a wave of terror through me. I felt my body shudder as the energy of the words shot right up through my spine. I heard the nurse say to my friend, *'Your results are negative, but I'm afraid your friend's are positive... She's pregnant.'*

In that moment, as fear rose from my belly and the blood coursed through my veins, my instincts told me that my life was about to take a profound turn and change me, and my heart, forever.

The shock had instantly hit my body. Time seemed to slow down and speed up simultaneously. The room was spinning and I felt faint. My body felt contracted, tight, restricted, blow after blow hitting the pit of my stomach and my throat. The overwhelm felt claustrophobic as my throat tightened and I could hardly catch a breath.

I wanted out of the room... out of my body, to breathe... to scream, to let the anger show that was bubbling up from deep inside of me and finally to let those tears flow. I felt my heart cry out...

Why me???

It felt like I was being airlifted out of my body and I was looking down on myself and the others in the room. I had literally checked out. Out of body, out of mind and I was floating. Hearing only the faint sound of the nurses voice in the background advising me on what next steps to take.

I'd entered into a state of denial, disbelief and complete dissociation, the last residues of trauma only leaving my entire system as I write these words today. It took days for me to pluck up the courage to tell my boyfriend. I had so much fear in me and felt paralysed inside.

I was in turmoil, and after much soul searching, I made a difficult decision to terminate my pregnancy, despite my deeply rooted Irish Catholic beliefs.

I had so many limiting beliefs ingrained in me at the time: religious, racial, cultural, societal and generational. I carried so much weighted shame and guilt around sex and pregnancy outside marriage, as well as mixed-race relationships. Of course, this wasn't always verbalised but I was very aware it existed.

Contraception was never discussed at home, as my mother had her own subconscious distorted beliefs and trauma, which like most of that generation had never been healed or acknowledged as significant for future generations.

So many stories left untold…

Abortion had not yet been legalised in Ireland so I had to travel to the U.K. with my boyfriend and a brother whom I was close to at the time. The day before the procedure, whilst alone in our accommodation, I asked the Divine for a sign to confirm I was making the right decision. Almost instantly, I felt movement in my belly for the first time, like butterflies or a somersault.

Overwhelmed with love from the energy emanating from my womb, I questioned why I was experiencing this now, after already committing to my decision and making arrangements. I'd come all this way…

Yet, I sensed a comforting guidance, a sense of love, protection and assurance that whatever choice I made, I was being led in the right direction.

Channelled Message

As I write this story from my 18-year-old self, I received an unexpected channelled message from spirit baby... which blew my mind.

'Siobhan, go make waves in the world. This is part of the process of divine reclamation. Your journey toward womanhood and empowering a nation betrothed to anger and irreverence. This is the journey to your heart, my child, lost and stolen on your journey into lifeform. You were never meant to fit in, and you were meant to stand out. Out from the masses, the crowds that say change is irreverent. You are the creator of your own being, master of your own mind, and you behold the qualities that make your right to thrive a divine reclamation.

A life of mediocrity awaits you if you bring this pregnancy to full term. This pregnancy is here only to show you the way, to carve the pathway. It's here to light the divine inside of you, to awaken the darkness of generational trauma, and bring light back to women and humankind.

You are carving a pathway into divine love, light, peace, and reverence. This is your heart, the journey to your soul, destiny, and unity.'

This is self-love.

And in that moment, I realised there was much more at play... this journey was so much bigger than me.

After the termination mixed emotions of relief, grief, self-expansion, almost elation moved through me. I felt accepted, guided and loved in those moments.

After I returned to Ireland, back to reality and into a very different cultural energy, things started to change in my relationship. I shut down. I felt myself spiral into an underworld of what I now know to be self-abuse, self-torture and self-loathing. I'd lost my way... and we separated a year or so after.

My health started to deteriorate on all levels and it wasn't long before the first patch of psoriasis appeared. Unknowingly, by breaking the chains of guilt, shame and repression, I found myself caught in a four-year cycle of disconnection, self-neglect and self-punishment. However, this was the path my soul needed to take, leading to a whole new chapter in my story. My mother had become pregnant at 17 and married my father. She had four children by the time she was 22. I'm the fourth child of 11. I wasn't going to do the same.

Then that's another story to tell...

This marked the beginning of my journey into ancestral healing, reclaiming body autonomy and the freedom to choose without shame or guilt. I wasn't born with the freedom to choose as part of my core beliefs and value system but I've now made it my top value in life, along with authenticity and integrity.

Breaking Chains

Freedom, authenticity and integrity.

From my own experience and daily practice, I've seen how cultivating deep body love and confidence through sensual and sexual arts helps us reclaim sovereignty and reconnect with our bodies, liberating our authenticity, our true erotic innocence. Our journeys aren't linear; they're multi-dimensional and through my work, personal healing and spiritual development, I've witnessed firsthand how perpetuating dysfunctional patterns of living and loving greatly impact our current lives and relationships. These are often rooted in unconscious, unresolved past life and ancestral trauma.

In 2010, when physical illness brought me into the magical world of energy healing and subconscious mind programming, the significance of generational healing in reclaiming our sensual and sexual health was fully awakened in me. I realised the profound opportunity we now have as women to take a stand and dismantle generational trauma and outdated patriarchal belief systems. As we grow, nurture and birth generation after generation, we hold the power within to break these chains and usher in a new era of empowerment and authenticity.

As a devoted mother, I'm committed to breaking these cycles so that my children and I can fulfil our souls potential and contribute to the exciting evolutionary shift happening right now on our planet. This ensures that future generations do not perpetuate these old ways of living and loving. I witness these incredible transformations daily in my own children, and I feel grateful to be on this path of unity and integration.

I believe empowering women's rights to full body autonomy is key and begins with women supporting women in unconditional love and acceptance, lighting the way in love and grace. What's right for one woman's soul experience isn't for another's and I believe it's imperative for women to create space for other women to move through their experiences safely, rather than repress them in guilt and shame. When the latter happens, old ways are perpetuated and we make little progress toward healing, autonomy and unity. Women have become the wayshowers and changemakers and must stop fighting each other at every corner. It's time to wake up to their old cycles, beliefs and values and intuit whether these systems still serve them and future generations.

Compassion, empathy and unity are essential parts in evolving our New Earth energy, as is healing the generational bloodlines for our children, those who've gone before us and for future generations to come. I didn't have the awareness or resources I needed at 18 years of age so I subsequently unconsciously repeated patterns, through that four-year cycle.

If my mother or I knew then what I know now, things would have been very different. In hindsight, my journey and evolution has allowed me to see that, during that four-year period, my decisions and experiences were not just based on the current situation at that time but also related to generational, past life trauma and soul contracts.

Let your Sensual Soul Shine

So what does it mean to let your sensual soul shine?

Sensual soul shine is that bright light, deep inside us, that ignites the senses, awakens the spirit, and invites us to embrace and live our very existence... empowered with an innate sense of purpose, passion, pleasure, aliveness and reverence. It reminds us of who we truly are at a heart and soul level, embracing the beauty and complexity of the human experience, and allowing us to revel in the inherent sensuality of that experience, as we journey deeper into our unique world of self-discovery.

True fulfilment arises from honouring the sacred union of our physical desires and our deepest soul yearnings. When we immerse ourselves in the pleasure of touch, taste, scent, sound and sight, being fully present in each moment, we really celebrate the fullness of life and all life has to offer us. We revel in the beauty of nature, feeding and nurturing the soul, savouring each magical moment with childlike wonder, in awe and with gratitude.

We embrace our shadows and light, honouring every aspect of our being with compassion and acceptance. We open to true intimacy, which begins with self-intimacy, tenderness, and self-connection.

This involves exploring our authentic desires, fears and vulnerabilities, shedding societal expectations with courage, compassion and self-acceptance, and embracing our authenticity... our unique beauty and truth. We reclaim our power, pleasure, passion and purpose, stepping into our truest selves and shining brightly.

We understand that basking in the glow of our sensual and sexual pleasure and all of its aliveness IS our birthright! We understand the significance of prioritising and cultivating more pleasure in our bodies as we know this supports its innate ability to heal, nurture, nourish and restore itself physically and emotionally, fostering better mental agility and spiritual union. A healed and regulated nervous system is the foundation for holistic health and vitality.

Inspiring New Ways of Living and Loving

Love making becomes a full body and soul sensual experience. The sensual soul honours the sacredness of sexual union as an alchemical pathway to spiritual awakening, sensual illumination and personal transformation. It transcends physicality, celebrating the divine within ourselves and our intimate partners, liberating us in ecstasy and bliss.

It fosters deep connection and mutual respect. It is ultimately a profound and satiating journey of higher love, unity and reverence, enticing and magnetising to us an open invitation to see the beauty and divinity in all that exists. Ultimately, sacred sensuality and sexuality is a path of awakening and enlightenment.

This journey is about enjoying the richness and sweetness of life to the fullest... admiring nature's beauty, tasting delicious food, feeling the warmth of the sun on our skin, star gazing in the night sky, and getting lost in the rhythm of the ocean.

Childhood memories... innocence, giggles, erotic tingles, curiosity and playfulness. Exploring our senses... hide and seek... hearts pounding... intuitive hits... listening with razor sharp ears... Hot sand between our toes at the beach... warm breeze... birdsong... children's cheers. Walking barefoot on the grass, morning dew, enlivening and inspiring...

Long hot summers immersed in nature's bliss, her womb... her creative power... her yoni... open to life and its aliveness. Making mud pies... squelching, satisfying... that felt sense between little fingers and toes, bringing feelings of contentment and assuredness, groundedness and control. Unifying that sense of belonging and peace.

This sensual soul journey is about appreciating every moment and feeling grateful for the wonder of being alive and in love with life. Remembering this through the eyes of a child but with wisdom of life experience and the divine mind.

About Siobhan Gannon

Siobhan Gannon is a holistic life coach specialising in the areas of energy healing, soul guidance and somatic sex and relationship coaching. Her business is Embodied Soulful Living and with over 15 years' experience in the holistic health field, she's trained in a multitude of modalities, each bringing its own unique magic to her ever evolving wellness toolkit! Based in scenic Connemara, Co. Galway, Ireland, Siobhan is a solo mom to three amazing young adults.

Siobhan's own journey through chronic illness and burnout has fuelled her commitment to prioritising pleasure and healing. Over the last 15 years, she has embraced her healer's path, gaining wisdom, faith and trust. Drawing from personal and clinic experiences, she provides safe, compassionate support to women facing transitional challenges such as menopause, abortion, divorce, single parenting, fertility issues, pregnancy and birth trauma, chronic stress, sexual health, relationships, and generational trauma.

Siobhan is not only committed to personal transformation but is also a passionate leader and advocate for healthy sex education. She has recently launched 'Enlightenment in the Bedroom' in Ireland, an Australian franchise, devoted to fostering open, healthy, body positive conversations around sex, pleasure, intimacy, and relationships. These live events for singles and couples aim to challenge societal taboos, shed light on generational trauma and outdated patriarchal belief and value systems and cultivate healthy relationships.

Passionate about women's empowerment and bridging spirituality, sensuality and sexuality, Siobhan guides clients on a journey of illumination and alchemy, transforming challenges into courage, confidence, clarity, and unshakeable trust. She combines the Akashic Records with somatic self-pleasure practices to facilitate healing and manifestation, empowering clients to embrace their psychic senses, natural sensitivity, sensuality and embody the vibrant souls they are here to be.

She's currently channelling her passion into writing her first book and oracle deck, both geared towards empowering women to live in their authentic aliveness.

Website: https://embodiedsoulfulliving.com/

'I suddenly understand that the reason other people, especially women, get upset with me "standing out" is because they work so very hard to blend in. It is not that I work hard at standing out, just that they work so hard not to stand out.'

– Carrie Myers

MY SENSUAL CIRCLE
by Carrie Myers

One of the many reasons I wanted to explore and collaborate on *Sensual Soul Shine* is to find my sensuality, once again. I miss feeling sexy, desirable, and powerful in my feminine self. I feel I used to exude sensuality, embody the softness, and shine from my carnal *authenticity*. But once my husband started being sexually curious outside our marriage, I lost that fire, that feeling of longing and drive to be, well, sexually open, sensual, and curious within myself. I have lost the ability to trust and relax in sexual safety. I am guarded and almost rigid, leaving my sensuality in a void. I pay more attention to "am I" doing the right things, making the right noises, saying the right things, and am I good enough? I am too much in my head and not enough in my body, my being. I no longer just flow with my desire. I am stagnant in not feeling like enough for him. My weight gain has been a barrier and, I feel, I subconsciously gained the weight as a protective factor in my sensuality. As much as I despise the extended belly and thick thighs, I feel no motivation to change my body. Does it even matter anyway? (I was in the best shape of my life when he started cheating.)

I do not know how to fix this. I feel such a push-pull around my body constantly. I read. I listen. I pray. I meditate. I try to tell myself that I must believe in the sensuality of my authenticity once again, yet I still feel encapsulated in my detrimental self-talk and barriers. I am working on finding the peace within myself and his touch, trust within our connection and truth within myself. I want to reignite my *divine spark*.

I, now, also have a fear of being vulnerable. Is this the wounded feminine energy that is blocking my sensuality? How do I release these wounds and remind myself that I deserve to live in the fullness of my femininity? As I stand in front of my youthful self, I see her striving to be who she was, in complete transparency and authenticity, and asking me why she cannot still be who she was, who she is in her authenticity. I feel the pain of her trying to break free of her cage as others continue to put more locks on the bars. Some of those "others" include my shadow self, and my protective subconscious. The self that is overflowing in self-pity, loathing and fearful of others' rejection and judgment. What still haunts me deep inside?

When I was in fifth grade, me and a group of my closest friends were supposed to perform a play or dance, something like that. We decided to wear sundresses for this performance. I only had a few sundresses at the time, so I told the girls that I would wear my brown sundress, and they told me which color they would wear. The day of the performance came, and I had decided the night before to wear one of my mom's sundresses, which was red. I was so excited to wear my mom's red sundress and proudly showed up in class. Well... this did not go over well with one of our group members. Angrily, she berated me and shamed me for changing my mind. She had brought brown ribbons for my hair and now, I had messed everything up. I felt myself grow small, wanting to disappear into the walls. Funnily, we never even got to do our performance – I do not remember why, but I vividly remember the feeling that I was left with, to this day, for wearing the red dress.

What I came to realize, after all these years, was that red stands out more so than most other colors, and this felt threatening to her. It was never my intention to stand out, I just wanted to wear the red dress, because it was my mom's and she let me wear it. I feel that this girl, who I thought was a friend, really did not want me to get more attention than her, just because my dress stood out.

Flash forward to August 2022. I was at the beach with my daughter and two of her friends. We set up a hot pink cabana, because I could not resist purchasing the hot pink! As we scanned the beach, we could see all the blue fluttery canopies crowding the taupe, sandy landscape, then there is mine, the bright, hot pink cabana standing out, grabbing everyone's attention on the beach. My friend said, *"See, Carrie, you even stand out in the crowd on the beach!"* This made me chuckle. I never truly intentionally choose to stand out, I just really chose to purchase what I like, which was the *Hot Pink!*

This also brought me right back to the red dress. That is when I realized that I will and should continue to stand out, speak my truth and love who I am.

So how does me telling you about the red dress and hot pink cabana relate to my sensuality? I have been asking myself that also. But, maybe, it is an expression of my drive to live from my authenticity and not care what others think or how they feel about me. Maybe it is my unconscious need to just be who I want to be, meant to be and truly am. When I choose a dress or cabana, I choose what lights me up, what calls to me and never consider that it may stand out or capture someone's attention more than the cookie cutter, mindless manufactured and socially acceptable monotony that is in our world today. I have never been one to jump through hoops, follow the crowd and blend in, and I refuse to start to do that now. I suddenly understand that the reason other people, especially women, get upset with me "standing out" is because they work so very hard to blend in. It is not that I work hard at standing out, just that they work so hard not to stand out. Bam!! Boy, that has landed hard and heavy just now.

Now, I see why I am so hell bent on authenticity. It is because I have always just been me and that aspect of my personality has just thrown so many off, those that strive to blend in and do all they should do, and I effortlessly stand out just by being me! So, for the life of me, I cannot understand why someone would try so hard to be something they are not!

Now let us link it back with my current troubles with sensuality...

I feel it is because I feel I am not being authentic, and I am too in my head around sex that it is creating a barrier for me. I am no longer the woman who is in the moment and feeling all the feels and doing what I do. I am thinking about doing it all correctly and breathing just right and saying the right words and touching the right places. What once was just how I was, was squashed with infidelity and self-doubt and now I am questioning if I am *performing* in the right ways instead of just being passionate and real.

Did I just come full circle?

> 'Internal stories left to harden, become our truths
> and mold us into doubtful, resentful belief structures.'
> - James Allen, As a Man Thinketh

GRAB YOUR JOURNAL
by Carrie Myers

- What is the universal truth about your sensuality?

- When did you stop nourishing your power?

- How do you let your conditioning unfurl to find your authentic self?

- What "ideal woman" are you competing against?

- How were you taught to ignore your power, your body, your desires?

- What are your unspoken needs, desires, yearnings, "crawling out of your skin" pain, love, and passions?

- How do you plan to get reacquainted with your womanhood, your divine feminine and your sensual self?

- Do you feel ***sexuality*** and ***sensuality*** are the same or different?

- How has/does trauma affect your ***sensuality***? (I suggest seeking a great counselor)

- Do you harbor unspoken needs, desires, "crawling out of your skin" yearnings? How do you seek to claim these desires?

- How does your perception of your body impact your ***sensual self?***

- Where have societal expectations dimmed your passions and ***sensual self?*** Does this world, heavy on the linear, driven, divine masculine, squash the nurturing, loving, soulfulness of the divine feminine?

- How does movement feed into your ***sensuality?***

- How do we, as women, unfurl our social conditioning, our competition, and our grief to, once again, find our ***authentic and sensual selves?***

- What does ***sensuality*** mean to you?

- What drew you to ***Sensual Soul Shine?***

- What does getting back in touch with nature do for your ***sensuality?*** How does Mother Nature inspire you to go with the flow and be your authentic self?

- What messages did you receive about sex, ***sensuality*** and/or pleasure when you were growing up? How have they impacted you and how have you moved through them?

- How has the way you feel about your body shifted throughout your life?

- Have you hidden or been shamed when you presented your **sensual or sexual authenticity** to your partner, friend or even yourself? What have you done about it?

- Have you listened to and embodied the way of being a "good girl", never allowing yourself to venture into your natural sexual energy? How have you begun to listen to yourself?

- How do you get in touch with your body and what it needs and desires?

- Have you achieved or are you seeking connection with yourself? Your partner? Your inner goddess? Your self-worth? Your confidence? Joy? Fulfilment? Release?

- When you go out, do you feel sexy and confident in how you dress? How do you carry yourself? How do you interact with others? What is your self-talk as you decide what to wear?

- Do you take time to nourish and nurture yourself? Hot baths? Massages? All the self-care ways?

- Have you realized that you deserve pleasure and the safety to surrender to your partner?

- Have you allowed yourself to release rigidity and feel into your feminine flow?

- How do you welcome playfulness into your daily life? Your sex life?

- Have you taken your people pleasing ways into the bedroom?

- What would it feel like to dance naked in the moonlight or rain?

- What myths of **sensuality** do you want to rewrite?

- When, where and how did you last feel, act, live from your true sensual self?

- As a young girl, did you feel more feminine than you do now? Explain.

- Can you identify a specific time that you squashed your feminine to fit into the more masculine way of being?

- What is the patriarchy to you?

- Describe the world as if it were ruled by women? A Matriarchal Society...

- How has living more linear and goal oriented dimmed your creative, ***passionate feminine?***

- What does ***passion*** mean to you?

- What role does ***passion*** play in your life?

- How do you balance your feminine energy in the masculine world?

- Do you long for change to balance and reclaim the ***sensual/feminine*** within yourself? Your relationships? The world?

- Throughout history there have been masculine powers that intentional attempted to wipe out feminine knowledge, power, and strength. What does this say to you about the imbalance of the feminine energy of today?

- Looking back at your life, can you recognize a specific event that made you back away from your ***true sensual self?*** Where did trauma play a role in you being less feminine, less passionate, less sensual, in your life? How have you/are you working through this pain?

- Did someone urge you to hide your feminine because of jealousy? Fear?

- Describe your ***authentic, feminine, sensual self*** as if she did not have any boundaries, pain, or expectations from others?

- How is ***sensuality*** different from sexuality?

- When do you feel the most ***sensuous?***

- Describe your bedroom, office, bathroom, etc. if you had the perfect **sensual home** to fit your authentic sensual self?

- What would you want to read if you were trying to **reclaim your sensual self** after a trauma?

- How did your parents' relationship effect your **feminine roles** within a relationship? The world?

- If you were to balance the world within the masculine and feminine energies, what changes would you make?

- How can you ask, or demand, **more sensual experiences** in the bedroom?

- What routines, when you have the time, make you feel your most **beautiful, sensual self?**

- If you were to dress as your **authentic sensual self,** what would you wear? What is stopping you from doing this every day?

- What would you tell your daughter about living in her **true feminine power?**

- Imagine a world where there were never witch hunts and fears around **feminine knowledge and power.** What would that world look like?

- What rituals do you have when you want to feel your **most sensuous?**

- Where, in nature, would you feel the ***most sensual?***

- If ***sensuality*** were the weather, what would the forecast be?

- How will you impact your friends as you ***reclaim your feminine power and sensuality?***

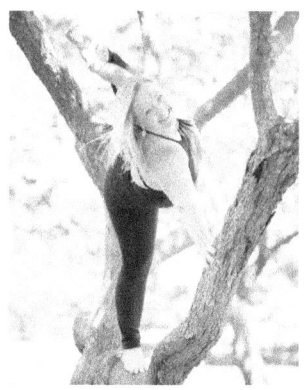

About the Lead Author

Carrie J. Myers, MSW, RYT 500, author, poet, program developer, speaker, wife, mother, and grandmother, has been writing since she was 10 years old. Her poetry, which reflects the phases of her life, has helped her process her journey along the way. As a yoga instructor, she discovers new ways to dig deep into her subconscious, pulling from her practice, the words that hold higher meaning and growth. She hopes to inspire change in the hearts and souls of her readers, while holding space for each interpretation to resonate with each soul. Carrie is passionate about creating and recognizing the beauty in the mess that life can throw at us, at times. Her goal is to help readers to rediscover their authentic selves, revive, create, and excavate their light from within.

Carrie is also the author of *Soul Confetti: Celebrating Life's Lessons* and lead author for the collaborative book, *Soul Shine: Excavate Your Light and Claim Your Soul's Purpose*, and several collaborations, magazine articles, and blogs

For more from Carrie, visit her website carriemyersauthor.com.

@cjmyerspoet
@SoulShineUnbound
@bethesparkmovement
@YourSelfProgram

www.ingramcontent.com/pod-product-compliance
Lightning Source LLC
Chambersburg PA
CBHW072053110526
44590CB00018B/3151